In Praise of Ādyā Kālī

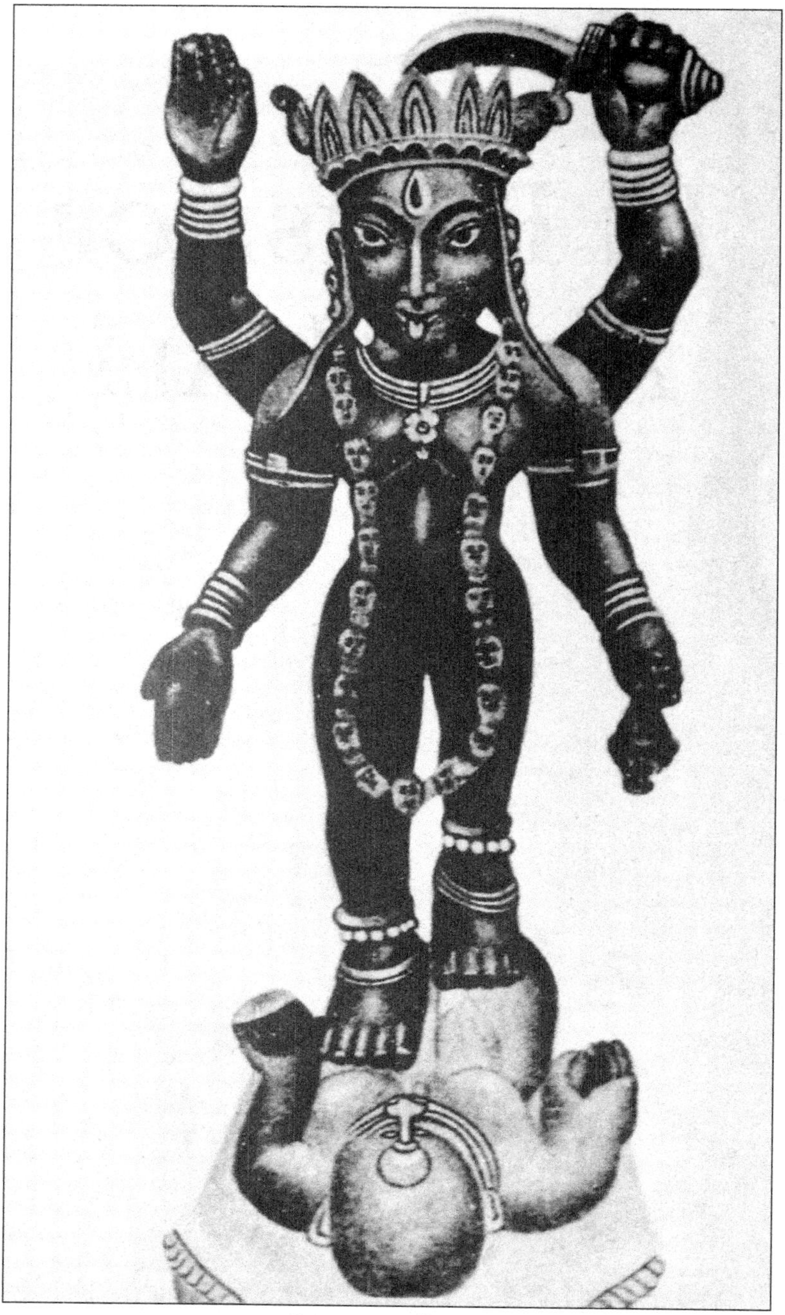

Oṁ namoḥ Ādyāye

IN PRAISE OF ĀDYĀ KĀLĪ

Approaching the Primordial Dark Goddess Through the Song of Her Hundred Names

Aditi Devi

HOHM PRESS
Chino Valley, Arizona

© 2014, Julia Aditi Jean

All rights reserved. No part of this book may be reproduced in any manner without written permission from the publisher, except in the case of quotes used in critical articles and reviews.

Cover Design: Zac Parker, Kadak Graphics, Paulden, AZ

Cover Image: Twenty-Armed Guhya Kālī. Vintage lithograph. Private collection. Used with permission.

Interior Design and Layout: Becky Fulker, Kubera Book Design, Prescott, AZ

Library of Congress Cataloging-in-Publication Data

Aditi, Devi (Ma).

In praise of Adya Kali : approaching the primordial dark goddess through the song of her hundred names / By Aditi Devi (Ma).

pages cm

Includes bibliographical references and index.

ISBN 978-1-935387-54-1 (trade pbk. : alk. paper)

1. Kali (Hindu deity)--Prayers and devotions. 2. Tantras. Mahanirvanatantra. Adyakalikadevyah satanamastotram--Criticism, interpretation, etc. I. Tantras. Mahanirvanatantra. Adyakalikadevyah satanamastotram. II. Title.

BL1225.K32A35 2013

294.5'211--dc23

2013030357

Hohm Press
P.O. Box 4410
Chino Valley, AZ 86323
800-381-2700
http://www.hohmpress.com

This book was printed in the U.S.A. on recycled, acid-free paper using soy ink.

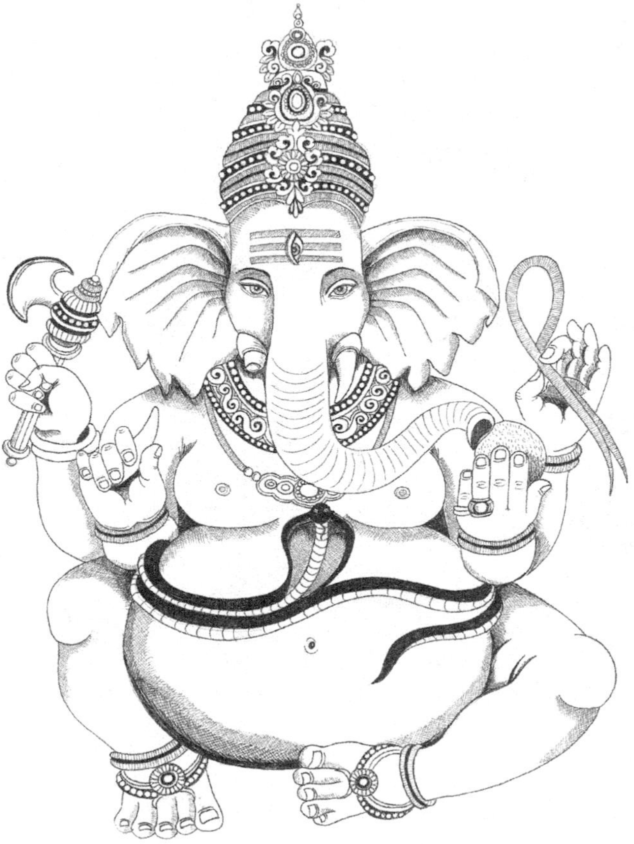

ॐ गं गणपतये नम
Oṁ gam Ganapataye namaḥ

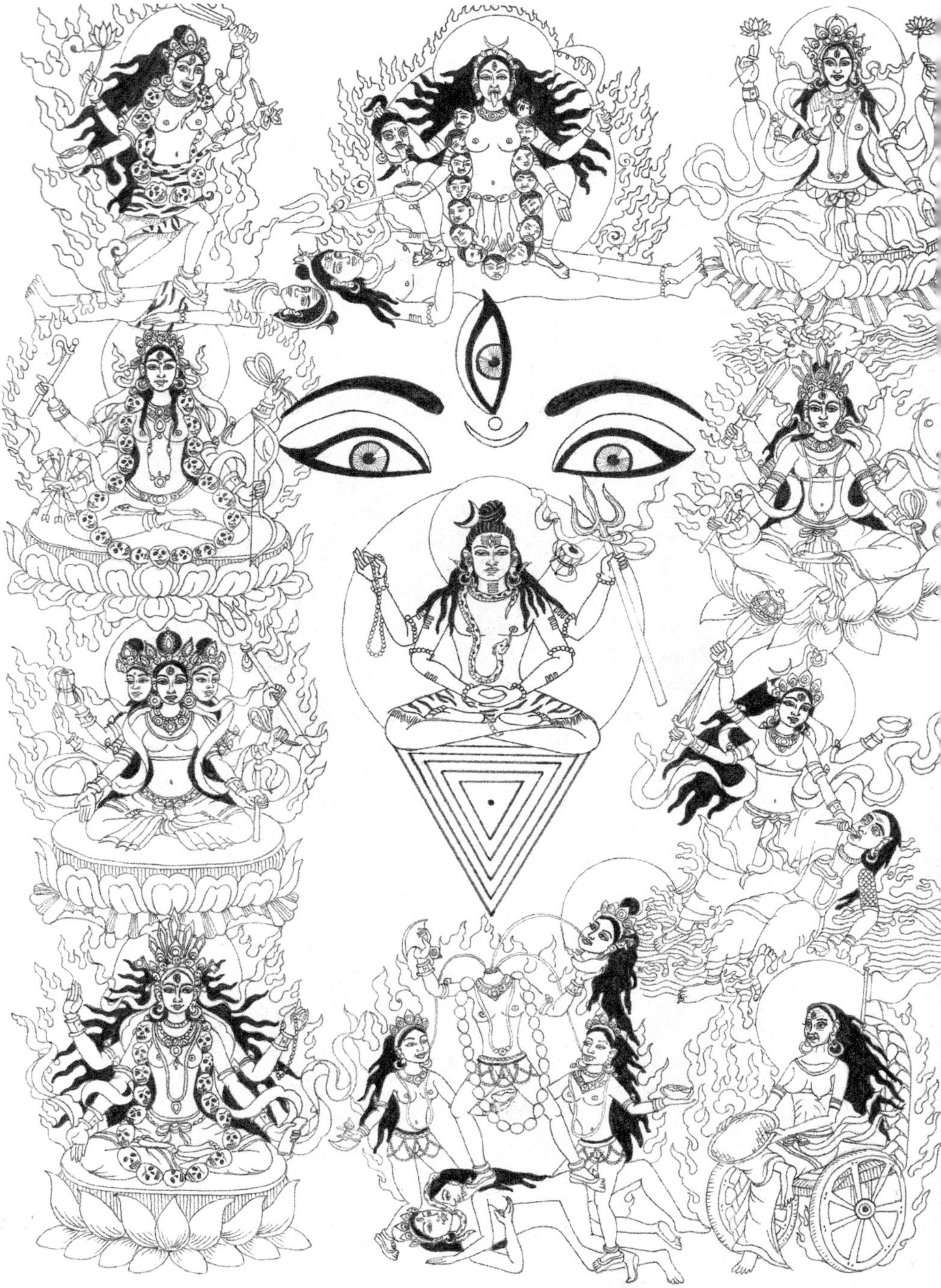

In front – She
To the left and
To the right – She
To the sides – She
Behind – She
In the lotus of the heart,
None other than She

On one road
And then the other
Wherever I turn,
There She Is

My suffering is of believing
She is distant
But there is no nature
Apart from Her

She She She She She She
What *is* this non-dualist creed
When She is all that Is?
(Amaruśatika; translated by Ina Sahaja, 2011)[1]

❀ ❀ ❀

Oṁ 64 Yoginīs,
Come here, come here!
(Rodrigues 2003:200)

Whether fierce or gentle, terrible to behold, all-powerful,
Residing in the sky, on earth, or in the vastness of space,
May these Yoginīs be well disposed towards me.

To those eternal Yoginīs by whose glory
The Three Worlds have been established,
To them I bow down, to them I pray.
(*Kulārṇava Tantra* 7.13 and 8.50, as cited in Dehejia 1986:34)

Contents

Foreword by Dawn Cartwright xi

I. Introduction 1

1. Her Names with Rose Petals 3
2. Kālī and Ādyā Kālī 8
3. The Turning Towards: Her Darkness and Her Fierceness 19
4. Śāktism, Śakti, and Tantra 32
5. The Kālīkula as Gynocentric and Womb-Centric 41
6. Śakti and the Yoni as the Primordial Matrix 47
7. Kālī's Tantras 57
8. Kālī's Names, Her Mantras, and the Nature of Transmission 61
9. How to Practice the *Song of the Hundred Names of Ādyā Kālī* 67

II. *Song of the Hundred Names of Ādyā Kālī* 81

III. Contemplations of Ādyā Kālī's Hundred Names 95

Acknowledgements 189

End Notes 195

Glossary 200

Bibliography 210

List of Illustrations 216

Index 218

About the Author 228

Contact Information 228

Foreword

by Dawn Cartwright

To look into the eyes of a Tantrika is to dance on the edge the cosmos.

Worlds and galaxies play along her lashes. Birth and death coexist—joyously—in the transparency of her gaze. Aditi Devi and I were presenting at a festival dedicated to the Divine Feminine in the spring of 2011, I turned a corner, our eyes met for the first time, I fell instantly in love.

As a teacher and seeker for many years along the Tantric path, I recognized this love immediately. I knew, simultaneously, I'd met a great adept, for only those who have died to all else can transmit the enormity of Kālī's love in a single glance. Aditi Devi is such a woman. The love recognized none other than Kālī.

In Praise of Ādyā Kālī: Approaching the Primordial Dark Goddess Through the Song of Her Hundred Names is this love affair. Rare and hidden traditions, enigmatic stories and detailed practices invite the reader to see, taste and touch Kālī themselves, in all her forms, sweet and terrible, as we are carried beyond words and descriptions into the living experience of the fierce mother goddess herself.

With tenderness and simplicity, the most intricate esoteric Tantrika practices are revealed, initiated, embodied. Aditi Devi initiates you, step by step into this ancient song in praise of

Kālī, revealing, in unexpected moments, the sublime within the mundane.

In my twenty-two years exploring the mysteries of Tantra and sexuality in my own practice, I've come to realize there comes a moment when skimming the surface no longer satisfies. *In Praise of Ādyā Kālī: Approaching the Primordial Dark Goddess Through the Song of Her Hundred Names* is a deep dive, it's Tantra in all its stark magnificence. The *Song of Her Hundred Names* has ignited all my practice and revealed to me a love that can be neither divided nor diminished.

Dawn Cartwright
Director Chandra Bindu Tantra Institute
August 10th, 2013
Santa Monica, California

www.dawncartwright.com

I.
INTRODUCTION

1

Her Names with Rose Petals

We are sitting knee to knee in the ritual space. There is a large shrine to several forms of Kālī in the center. Her name, her names, repeating Ādyā Kālī's names one after the other. Chanting them, singing them, relishing them, laughing with them, and crying with them, knowing that she is manifesting as the form of each and every one of her names. As each Sanskrit name moves through our bodies and mouths and is uttered into the space between us, we offer a rose petal to the one sitting across from us by touching it to our heart, throat, and then third eye before placing it at the feet of the form of Kālī as our friend. Here, in a circle of beloved yoginīs and yogis, we are reciting the *Song of the Hundred Names of Ādyā Kālī* during our weekly community Kālī *Pūjā*.* Everything changes as a result. Tensions have drained away and discomforts are forgotten. At some point, the room begins to glow as the recitation resonates and everyone begins to feel that their beloved Kālī is sitting knee to knee with them receiving their offering. We also begin to know that we are the form of Ādyā Kālī and a loved one is making offerings to us as we morph through all of her sacred forms. We were, and are, all that. Relationality is unfolding. The room is filled with rose petals, with her love, and with our devotion. Our love and awareness have moved out to meet her in each other.

* All terms marked with * are defined in the Glossary, pp. 200–210.

The version of our community recitation of the Tantric liturgy of the *Song of the Hundred Names of Ādyā Kālī* that you hold in your hands was first practiced inside this sacred *cakra** of female practitioners, yoginīs, who had requested that we undertake a community practice commitment based on my devotional re-translation and editing of the original Tantric liturgy of the *ādyā kālikādevyāḥ śatanāma stotram*. Together, we committed to the spiritual practice (*sādhana**) of the recitation of this ancient and sacred liturgy to the Śakta Tantric goddess Kālī over 108 nights during a recent cold and dark winter. We undertook a *saṅkalpa** together, a formal spiritual commitment to this precious Kālī sādhana.

This liturgy consists of the hundred names of Ādyā Kālī that begin with the first consonant of the Sanskrit alphabet, *ka*.[2] The names themselves are a sublime garland of flowers that we offer at her feet by reciting them out loud, one by one, in front of a shrine dedicated to Ādyā Kālī. This book, *In Praise of Ādyā Kālī*, is the form of and source of support for you in your relationship with Kālī and for the study, practice, and contemplation of the *Song of the Hundred Names of Ādyā Kālī*. Your devotion, curiosity, and willingness are all you need to begin. Here you will find instructions for building a shrine to Ādyā Kālī, developing a nightly spiritual practice that includes the contemplations focusing on each name; these can be used as a meditation in conjunction with undertaking a nightly recitation of the *Song of the Hundred Names of Ādyā Kālī*. Perhaps you might consider reciting this liturgy for 108 nights.

The commitment to recite her names is a potent form of spiritual practice, as our practice community discovered early in: we had undertaken a powerful form of spiritual practice both as individual devotees and as a community. Even though we were separated geographically, spread across the globe, we begin to have the experience of moving together in this, as one.

This community experience resonates with an important Tantric vow in the spiritual lineage of *Kālīkula*:* no one left behind. Practicing together is an inclusion of all forms of relationship. It is an inclusion of everyone and everything on the path. As you begin to consider doing this practice, please know that you are not alone. While you may not personally know others who are reciting the *Song*, I assure you that there are yoginīs and yogis all over the world who are doing this same practice right now. I also recite her *Song* daily. It is rich and powerful to do this together in community. It's also substantial to undertake this practice as an individual devotee, letting your own love affair with Kālī develop in the intimacy of this recitation of her hundred names.

In Sanskrit, the name of this Kālī liturgy is the *ādyā kālikādevyāḥ śatanāma stotram* and it comes from the *Mahānirvāṇatantraṃ* (more commonly referred to as the *Mahanirvana Tantra*). This liturgy is found in Chapter Seven of the *Mahanirvana Tantra* and is sometimes also called the *ādyākālī svarūpa stotram*. In English, this translates to the *Song of the Hundred Names of Ādyā Kālī* or the *Song of Ādyā Kālī's Own Form* pointing to a major theme: this song of Ādyā Kālī's names is her very form. In some of the English-language literature, this liturgy is also sometimes referred to as the *Tantrik Hymn to Kālī* or *The Hundred Names of Goddess Kālī*.[3]

This book is an offering of support for you in considering undertaking a more formal devotional relationship to Kālī as well as to support the development of your ability to move love and awareness (aka bliss and freedom) through an open body. This is the path of unfolding towards embodied awakening that is Kālī's lifeblood. While the original impetus for this devotional translation of Kālī's name liturgy and for the 108 night sādhana commitment was to fulfill this request of my female students, yoginīs, the recitation of this liturgy can be undertaken by anyone who has a hunger to dive profoundly into their relationship with Kālī. What this means is that the material in this book will have the flavor of the original teachings offered to a community of women; this is reflective of the philosophical and spiritual worldview of the northern Kālīkula (the details and nuances of what this means will unfold as we proceed). Everyone is welcome here even with this gynocentric focus.

In Praise of Ādyā Kālī is designed for a wide-ranging audience. As spiritual pilgrims, we are more highly educated and more widely traveled than ever. Our hunger for knowledge (and the availability of so much on the Internet) has enhanced our abilities to take in information that just a decade ago might have been reserved for conversations among elite scholars or whispered between esoteric practitioners in remote caves, forests, and godowns. Today, everywhere, people are hungry to touch the depths of beingness. I offer all of this fully, even if doing so may take us into the realm of the esoteric footnote to provide more depth of understanding for those who want and enjoy such things. Foreign language terms have been kept for the sheer beauty and precision of the words (and are often not able to be easily rendered into English). Long intricate definitions and complex philosophical discussions are included. There is an extensive glossary in the back to support you with the words in South Asian languages, including the diacritical marks, which may prove useful as your studies and experiences grow.[4] The bibliography is a bit much, I admit, yet perhaps you will add a few of the items listed to your own treasure box of wisdom. As astute readers with devotional yearnings, I trust you to take in what you want, and what serves you, and to leave the rest for another moment. Some of the most important books I ever read have challenged me to grow because they either acted as conveyors of a transmission, or they pushed up against the edges of my own intellectual or emotional boundaries inspiring me to keep going.

This book is dense in places and playful in others. My hope is that the threads of scholarly information, practice wisdom, and personal experience that are intermingled here will support you on your journey of increasing depth, devotion, and connection. May this liturgy in praise of Ādyā Kālī be an offering to you as you establish your own relationship to her. May all beings benefit! *Oṁ namoḥ Ādyāye!*

2

Kālī and Ādyā Kālī

What does this all mean and who is Kālī, more precisely? I have been sitting with the question of what can I share with you about my beloved, the love of my life. What can I say about her that will support you to know her? How do we slip into this river together, in a way that will help you approach the blue-black goddess Kālī at the center of the yoniverse? There is no way that I can fathom a simple introduction as I write this. I am thinking of all the practitioners that I know, and of how Kālī came to each of them in a flash, wild, uncontainable, fierce, penetrating, and unremitting. She has been known to come on as lightning: bold, loud, and crackling on a clear day, taking us to our knees. We then have to learn to make room for her in our lives, in our bodies, and then eventually learn to fall in love. There is not a straightforward way that this happens, nor a clear path.

To begin to offer a picture and hopefully thus a feel for a few of the threads that allow us to experience Kālī directly, here is a poem to the Kālī of the cremation grounds by Rāmlāl Dāsdatta of Bengal, in the style of the love poems to Kālī from her heartland.

Because You love cremation grounds
I have made my heart one
so that You

Black Goddess of the Burning Grounds
can always dance there.
No desires are left, Mā, on the pyre
for the fire burns in my heart,
and I have covered everything with its ash
to prepare for Your coming.
As for the Conqueror of Death, the Destructive Lord [Śiva],
He can lie at Your feet. But You, come, Mā,
dance to the beat; I'll watch You
with my eyes closed.
(McDermott 2001b:74-75) [5]

There are so many elements primary to Kālī in this poem: her presence with death—and her presence as death—in the cremation grounds; her unending dance which brings both life and death; the way she burns up all that separates us from her; the way she takes up residence in our bodies as a burning force, a fiery urgency that cannot be cooled; her love of ash and bones as a reminder of how short life is, how transitory our existence. Through her, we can come to know what is larger than our own life and death. We let so much die (or we burn it down in the middle of the night) so we might have room for her in our lives, for her union with Śiva (another life-death dancer). Śiva beats the drum, and is the dancehall. Kālī dances. We watch it all from the inside out with our eyes closed; we are making love to her and him, in our bodies, in the endless fires. Kālī is a mystery and also very plain. She is the transcendent cosmic birthing and the daily midwiving of life.

The renowned Bengali devotional poet Ramprasad Sen has described this aspect of her thus:

You are the mother of all
And our nurse. You carry the Three Worlds

In Your belly.
(Nathan and Seely 1999:16).

This womb-aspect of Kālī is ever present side by side with her cremation ground forms. She is also desire. Her flavors are endless.

Kālī is truly the love of my life. She is my beloved. My life is oriented to the rhythms she dictates, to the service she requests (and requires). Her holy days, her moons, her festivals. She entered my body more than twenty-four years ago and it took me a long time to come to terms with this; it was some time after that reckoning that I began the slow movement towards falling in love with her. For some time now, I have been totally and irrevocably in love with her. I know that my life, body, and being are not separate from union with her. It's not always pretty, nor is it easy. But it is rich and more fulfilling than anything else I've done.

Dedicating myself fully to serving her is the most interesting experiment I can run with my life. Even so, I don't expect anyone else to follow in my footsteps; please, know that your relationship with Kālī is on your terms. I'm at one wild end of the spectrum in terms of what is possible.

I encourage you to find your own way with this, with her. Especially since Kālī is a bit scary for some people. After seeing images of her, hearing stories, or strolling around the Internet, it seems that most of what we can find focuses on her frightening death-giving aspects, or is just plain confusing and without the necessary background material to make sense of this fierce dark esoteric Tantric goddess. One of the things that I love about Kālī is that she is also the life-giving and nurturing mother. Kālī is also a healer and protectress. She guards the doorway between the manifest and the unmanifest. She brings the unmanifest into form, and in this form, she is Ādyā Kālī, the primordial Kālī. Kālī is also a lover; and not surprisingly, she is the beloved. She is the heat of kuṇḍalinī. She is the fire pit, the fire, and the fire-tender. Kālī has so much strength and capacity that she can heal all our wounds and take away all our fears.

Not only is Kālī the darkness, but she eradicates darkness as well. She gives the disease and removes it. This is one of the great paradoxes of the fierce Tantric goddesses: they are the quality that they also heal. We walk towards her, and this, in order to be free of it. Kālī shows us the way to freedom. She is fierce, in many of her forms, and yet she also offers peace, truth, goodness, and beauty. All of these qualities are hers as well, and thus also available to us as her devotees. Can you feel how her darkness and fierceness might also be peace, truth, goodness, and beauty? What is this paradox that Kālī inhabits as her primordial nature?

Part of the beauty of the liturgy of Kālī's hundred names is that many of the names apparently contradict each other. Coming into relationship with this contradictory nature of Kālī (and thus all reality) allows us to practice into understanding how *all* aspects of existence are her. From here, we can begin to feel how our personal existence, *just as it is*, is her grace, her living embodiment. This is the mystery lived in full embodiment.

Underneath all of this is the understanding that our bodies, energies, bodily fluids, when combined with spiritual practices and devotion to Kālī, can lead us to awakening in this body, in this lifetime. Our bodies offer us all we need to move into union if we are willing to enter into this landscape wholeheartedly, with devotion, and continually asking if we can see goddess now. How about now? Is this Kālī? That? Yes, it's all Kālī. All of it. Working this conceptual edge along with the body refinements of spiritual practice can suffuse our awareness with these realizations, transform our molecular structure, and guide us into the fluidity that allows union in all forms.

Our daily Kālī practice is the centerpoint-*bindu** that takes us into our inner depths, establishes our relationship to her, and from that rich pulsation we emerge into relationality with others. This recitation of Kālī's hundred names is focused on moving outward from this bindu-center, from the depth of our personal practice, into relationality with others.

The *Song* that is the substance of this book focuses on the form of Kālī that we call *Ādyā Kālī*. This is the fiery graveyard Kālī and the cool loving Mother, both. Who, or what, then is Ādyā Kālī in this context? The term *Ādyā* means *primordial, primal, first, original,* or *archean*.[6] Ādyā Kālī is the primordial energy, *śakti*, that creates, preserves, and transforms/dissolves all existence. At times, in some sources, Ādyā Kālī is understood to be identical with Dakṣiṇkālī, the four-armed form of Kālī who first entered my body back in the day many years ago on the edge of the Kathmandu valley at one of her open air shrines.

As the primordial śakti, Ādya Kālī is sometimes also called *Ādyā Śakti*. In this form, she is the primordial energy of the cosmos and the female energies of creation. She is ultimate reality and non-dual union, to use another vocabulary. She is pure consciousness and bliss, intermingled, before manifestation. Of course, in this primordial state before manifestation, there is no gender. Gender requires form. Before form manifests, it is pure potential. We refer to this energy of potentiation as feminine, she, because it has the power to produce, it has the power to give birth to form. Thus Ādyā Kālī is the womb of all creation. In this worldview, from the point of view of those who worship Kālī, she is also known as *Brahman** and this is made even clearer by some of the references to her as Kālī-Brahman. Another of Kālī's epithets is Brahmamayī, meaning "She Whose Essence is Brahman" (McDermott 2001b:173). Ādyā Kālī is Brahman, ultimate reality, inseparably.

Since Ādyā Kālī herself has no physical form, at least in the primordial state of Brahman, there are very few statues or representations of her. One of the two rare depictions of her

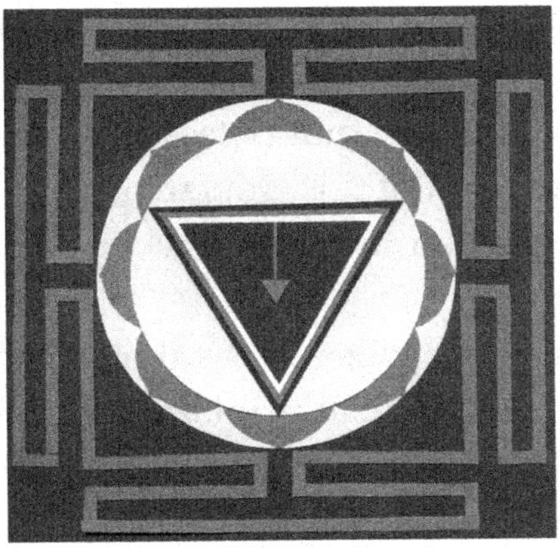

One version of a Yoni Yantra

is as a doorway or portal. This is the doorway between the manifest and the unmanifest. Another manifestation is as the squatting goddess who is sometimes called Lajjāgaurī; this form emphasizes her birthing of the cosmos from her body, her form.[7] She is both the static and the vibration as well as the formless as it gives form. She is the cosmic primordial womb, the *yoni**-matrix of existence, the yoniverse itself. Artistically, Ādyā Kālī is thus also sometimes represented as a *yoni-yantra** or just the yoni (womb and external genitalia). She is the threshold between formless and form, and between the unmanifest and the manifest. In addition, it could be said that Ādyā Kālī gives birth to the other forms of Kālī that we might know as Mahākālī or Dakṣiṇkālī.

How does the formless give birth to the form of all existence? This formless Ādyā Śakti becomes the universe first through a glimmer of light:

> She is light itself
>   and transcendent
> Emanating from Her body are rays
>   in thousands, millions, hundred millions.

There is no counting their great numbers.
It is by and through Her that all things
moving and motionless shine.
It is by the Light of this Devi that
all things become manifest.[8]

This *body* that is described in the third line is her light body, her womb body, her original primordial form. She is this light manifesting all of this existence as we know it. Her light permeates this world we know (as does her darkness, which we will discuss a little later on).

After her light, the next movement towards form is the formation of the *tattva*.* As one author describes it, "The term [tattva] is derived from the root *tat* meaning 'that' which is an epithet of *brahman*, the ultimate reality" (Bhattacharyya 2002:163). Here we feel more of the tendrils of connection that are held within Ādyā Kālī: ultimate reality (Brahman), the womb, and the manifestation of the tattvas from light. The tattvas unfold light into form. The thirty-six tattvas thus manifest from the womb mother of all existence.

One way that the term tattva can be translated is as *fundamental*; and in this system there are at least thirty-six fundamental building blocks of manifest existence. Kālī is here in the tattvas, linking them all together in her body. A tattva is an *element* or aspect of manifest existence that comes forth from the formless deity into concrete manifestation. Examples of tattvas in manifestation include earth, water, fire, air, ether, what we know as the senses (the mediums for olfactory sensations, taste sensations, visual sensations, etc.), excretion, sexuality, movement, apprehension/understanding, speech; locomotion is her tattva too. There is a great list of the tattvas on Wikipedia should you feel like getting even more esoteric. Ādyā Kālī brings forth the thirty-six tattvas so that existence and our embodied experience of existence can take form. One of the forms this takes is actually you. Imagine her birthing all aspects of you.

Another way to understand this is that the tattvas manifest as each of her names as elucidated in the *Song of the Hundred Names of Ādyā Kālī*. Each of these forms has a distinct, unique flavor and the entire list of her names encompasses all of existence. While all these forms are indeed part of Ādyā Kālī's being, they are not her entirety. How could they be? How can this primordial ultimate non-dual reality have a singular all-inclusive form? One way to approach this question is to begin to take in the depth and complexity of Ādyā Kālī's forms through the recitation of her hundred names that begin with *ka*. In this way, we can begin to have the direct experience of her, the felt experience of her, in our bodies and around us. This, by the way, is the essence of why we undertake pilgrimage: to feel her body in the landscape, temples, and people and let it permeate us.

On endless pilgrimage to all the forms of her body that I can find, I was directed towards her formless form by a devotee while on a trip to Kolkata. He insisted on showing me one of Mā's sacred outdoor Tantric shrines as well as pointing me towards the hidden jewel of a temple called Ādyā Pīṭh that is her formless self (http://www.adyapeath.org). It is hidden around the back ways near the Dakṣiṇeśwar Temple for Mā Kālī on the Hooghly River.[9] Here, next to an orphanage, in the back alleys, is the seat/place/abode of Ādyā, the formless Primordial She. The temple is richly intertwined with the lives and spiritual devotion of the famous saint Śrī Rāmakṛṣṇa, his wife Śrī Śāradā Devī, and one of Rāmakṛṣṇa's disciples Annada Thakur.[10] This large and airy temple complex is a shrine to ultimate reality as Kālī and it is also a remembrance of her form as ultimate reality.

As the temple is open for *darśan** for only a few minutes each day, we sat at the viewing platform which is perched across the way from the main Ādyā Pīṭh temple. This was the closest that we could get to the temple and it is the closest that most devotees and visitors can get. Primarily only the priests go up on the temple platform, and only the priests are allowed inside the main temple. Sitting on the cool cement, pressed in tightly in the women's section, I gazed at the enormity of a temple that felt in this moment somehow distant. I had grown accustomed to the intimacy of the Kāmākhyā Temple in Assam, one of my spiritual homes, where we come into direct full-bodied contact with the goddess Kāmākhyā Mā. As I sat at Ādyā Pīṭh I questioned: Why would they build a temple in such a way as to keep us so far separated from her?

When the immense doors of the temple finally opened, there was an audible gasp and murmurs of "*Mā*" moved through the crowd. I was struck by the enormity of the shrine and of her in this moment. The impact of her presence on my physical and subtle bodies gave me insight as to why she was so far away; I might have been disintegrated by her presence had I been much closer!

I also understood viscerally how Ādyā Kālī is so vast and so immense that she cannot be contained by structures. With the three-story-tall doors flung wide open, she was bursting out and flowing towards us and through us. She was all existence moving. All that I was feeling and seeing in that moment was her presencing for our benefit. Like a tsunami, Ādyā Kālī rolled through us on the platform across the way. I was swamped by her full presence; how could I ever have thought I was separate? I drank her in with every breath and as nourishment to my entire body on all the levels.

Across the way, inside the temple, the *mūrti** has three levels. At the base is a large image of Śrī Rāmakṛṣṇa. As the founder of the famous Dakṣiṇeśwar Temple to Kālī, he is quite famous and revered as a great Indian saint. In this neighborhood, he is the guru of all and everything, the guru of ultimate reality. Above him is an equally large image of what they call Ādyā Mā. She is standing and striding forward towards us, her devotees. This is the same form as the goddess Dakṣiṇkālī and is of course related to the main form of Kālī at the Dakṣiṇeśwar Kālī Temple.

Above them, at the top level, is a mūrti of Rādhā-Kṛṣṇa; they are so close to each other that it took my breath away. The lovers intertwined atop Ādyā Kālī's head. Is this what she dreams of at night? Is this her daily visualization upon arising? Is this how she understands all reality?[11] Inside of Kālī's primordial womb we find the guru, this primordial Kālī (as Dakṣiṇkālī), and the union of Rādhā and Kṛṣṇa. Again, the union just springs up all around, in all forms, winding up into itself, in every way.[12]

That Kālī has this transcendent nature, is this transcendent nature, can be found in the oldest written documents, the oldest Tantras, that mention Kālī worship. She is *That* from the beginning of our documented sources and is the primordial womb. This Tantric text, the *Yonigahvara* (*Recess of the Womb*), dating from about 1200 C.E. relates that she is: ". . . beyond the senses, inconceivable, of free volition, free from defects, identical with the stainless supreme sky . . . [residing in] the sphere beyond the sky . . . " (Goudriaan (1981:76). Ādyā Kālī, thus, is nondual love-awareness, the sphere, or bindu, moving as consciousness in the primordial womb and taking form so that we might be in relationship with her. She is truly the mother of the universe and thus also the mother of enlightenment. The mother of everything, really.

Ādyā Kālī has a special place in north and northeastern India, where her devotees are numberless and her forms are endless. This Kālī is the primordial matrix of ultimate reality. She is the field of all. She is Śakti. She moves all that is unmanifest into manifestation. She is primordial reality. She is all that is, was, and will ever be. She is the amorphous Kālī who then takes shape through our recitation of her mantras and her names. She is the primordial womb mother, the birthing goddess, and the hag-crone. All faces, all bodies, all forms are hers. Nothing left out.

A website dedicated to the Ādyā Pīṭh (Ādyā Peath) Temple includes photos as well as audio downloads of the *Ādyā Stotram* and her mantras (http://www.adyapeath.org/Docs.html). The *Ādyā Stotram* includes praise to Kāmarūpa, Kāmākhyā, the womb-yoni goddess of Assam. The pieces of my love affair with Kālī coalesce here in her primordial womb: Dakṣiṇkālī, Ādyā Pīṭh, Dakṣiṇeśvar, Rādhā-Kṛṣṇa, Kāmākhyā, and Gurvī*-Guru:* not separate, not separate.

3

The Turning Towards: Her Darkness and Her Fierceness

As we explore her mysteries as the play of light manifesting through the primordial womb, you may begin to understand as well that Kālī is associated with the deep and fecund dark. In alignment with this, she is often blue-black in color, and this distinctive coloring is often mentioned in descriptions of her. She is called *Dark Devī* (Nathan and Seely 1999:9, 19).

This darkness of hers is not something to be pushed away or held at arm's length. Kālī's primordial darkness is part of what takes form through the recitation of the *Song of Her Hundred Names*. For example, one description of her from the *Song* is as Kālarātriḥ, She Who Is the Night of Darkness. Another name is Kādambinī, She Who Is as Dark as a Bank of Rain Clouds.[13] As such, Kālī asks us to come to terms with her darkness, and thus all forms of darkness, in ourselves and the world. There is fecundity and hope and love in this darkness as we see in these descriptions of her that remove our fears: "Your name can blot out the fear of Death," (Nathan and Seely 1999:16) or

> Remembering that Her feet
> Cancel all fear,
> Who needs to fear Death?
> (Nathan and Seely (1999:53)

The final line of the *Song of the Hundred Names of Ādyā Kālī* points to this as well: "I make obeisance to She Who Is . . . the Destroyer of the Fear of Death." Her darkness has the power to remove all of our fears; her darkness is the remedy. Her darkness is also the spiritual path. As Andrew Schelling articulates so well in his description of fierce imagery found in the devotional poetry to Kālī: "This image, ghastly to those unschooled in its hidden meanings, holds precise philosophical and tantric instruction" (Schelling 2011:233). Holding this understanding close will support you as you practice the *Song of the Hundred Names of Ādyā Kālī*. The remembrance that there is wisdom and spiritual instruction to be found in all the forms of the dark is a profound teaching.

We tend to live in a world that valorizes the light over the dark in so many ways. One of the common (mis)understandings found in the spiritual teachings available to us in the West these days is that spiritual development means ascending, moving towards the light, and being light: We move upwards and out as a form of spiritual development. Let us explore another view here, the view that is central to the Kālī Practices and the Kālīkula.

That first autumn, when the original community of yoginīs committed to the *Song of the Hundred Names of Ādyā Kālī*, many of us were in parts of the world where the daily amount of sunlight was decreasing. Many of us, consciously and unconsciously began to focus on ways to increase the light in our lives as the natural darkness moved towards us and through us. I offered the yoginīs these same instructions around transforming their relationship to the dark (both the external darkening of the season as well as Kālī's darkness). Part of my own spiritual training has been to constantly *move towards* that which we perceive and experience as dark and constricted: moving into the dark whenever possible is to meet the darkness (and everything) with love, openness, and availability. We don't try to counteract the dark by increasing the light, instead, we sit with what is actually happening whether it is the increasing dark or the increasing light.

My training and experience teaches that aligning with the dark as a source of wisdom is a vital part of the path of the yoginī and yogi; it is essential to who we are in these bodies. Making friends with the dark, our dark, her dark, is part of the path of embodiment. If you don't have experience with welcoming the dark, or if you have been enculturated or trained to avoid the dark, I'm inviting you to transform that here with your recitations of the *Hundred Names of Ādyā Kālī*. It is a real opportunity we have to befriend ourselves and her. This practice, and other practices in the Kālīkula, focus on bringing the energies down into our bodies, into form, in the pelvis. We come into embodiment and relationship with all sensation as the divine, as spirit.

Let me explain simply: she is the dark. All of her qualities and forms that are listed in the *Song of the Hundred Names of Ādyā Kālī* are her dark form coming into manifestation. The gift of the dark is union with her, in all her forms, in all forms, in all manifest and unmanifest existence. All of this exists within ourselves as well. Instead of turning away from the dark, the shadow, the scary, and the wounded, we turn towards it knowing it is a fertile source of wisdom and teaching.

Our nightly practice, of the *Song of the Hundred Names of Ādyā Kālī*, with a focus on one of her names, supports us in generating a kind of relaxed ease and awareness in our bodies/minds/spirits and with the dark as Kālī. We rest in her flow. In addition to linking our bodies and beings to Kālī, it also supports us in generating love and awareness. This allows me to be aware of myself, as Aditi Devi, and aware of something happening that is called Aditi Devi. There is spaciousness and a simultaneous dual awareness. I am both feeling something (feeling my body, my emotions, my relationships, my environment) and I'm also able to gain a little perspective and see myself in it. One teacher describes this as being in the room and watching the room simultaneously. Both perspectives are valuable.

Once we have developed this dual sense of awareness of ourselves, we are ready to move towards a richer world of practice. When we know that we can return again and again to a knowing of our own inner world (subtle body and all that is there) as well as an awareness of ourselves in space and time, when we have allowed a sense of curiosity to develop around the experiences of others instead of an instant reactivity, it is time to go further into our practice. You may not yet be ready to do this, and that's just fine. I bring it to our conversations here, though, so we know what we are moving towards and cultivating. This deepening involves the practice of turning towards constriction and closure with openness. Let me repeat that in a slightly different way. When we feel constriction, in ourselves or in others, we practice to turn towards it with love and openness: *turn towards with openness and availability*. This means moving outside of ourselves at the moment when we want to constrict and turn inwards and separate out. All of us know what the quality of closure feels like; it is what creates disconnect and separation. It is actually pain and suffering. We may close in order not to feel the suffering of others, or to distance ourselves from our own pain. Or perhaps it is just an old automatic response to our own pain, and to the pain and suffering of others. We may never have trained in openness nor been in a context that valued it. Yet, we can feel the beauty of openness in others and we can feel the magnetic pull of it. We are actually drawn towards openness in others, even if we can't source it on our own. Right now, can you think of someone you know who exudes an openness that you enjoy, that you can relax into?

Whatever the underlying reasons for our habits of closure, our practice with Kālī allows us some of the love, space, and freedom to begin to relate to ourselves and the world differently. In many Tantric lineages, we even take a vow about this: it is one of the first and most fundamental vows we can take on the path. We vow to practice turning towards constriction with openness. The vow doesn't mean we get it right, but it serves as an orienting compass as we move through our lives. This is a vow that we break constantly, actually, and yet return to as much as possible.

I'm not asking, nor even suggesting, that you take this on as a vow. I'm mentioning the vow only to give you a sense of what a serious piece of business this is, how seriously Tantric practitioners take this practice of turning towards closure with openness.

Would you like to run a small experiment with this in your life? If so, perhaps you would like to consider the following questions for yourself: Can you identify someone you have in-person contact with who exudes a quality of openness? If so, see if you can identify what it is about their openness that attracts you, and note if you simultaneously have any negative associations or feelings about their openness? Do you judge it either negatively or positively? Do you shut down in this person's presence? Do you tell yourself any stories about this openness? Can you feel their openness as a quality in your own body? What does it feel like? Can you magnify this? Do you want more of it or less? Why?

As a second step in this experiment, which can be done at the same time as you address the questions above, in your daily devotion of reciting Kālī's names, bring your awareness to your own experience in such a way that you become aware of ease, freedom, and love inside yourself. You are feeling these qualities, you are these qualities, and you are aware of them in yourself, moving through you, as you. Can you, perhaps, with the help of Kālī's names, expand those qualities outwards at all? To the edges of your own skin? Out beyond your skin? Can you engage with others with these qualities moving through you? Perhaps you can identify some place in your life that has some closure in it and practice turning towards it with openness, for just this week? It doesn't have to be anything big; just something near that you could work with easily. What might that be like? How might this practice change something in your life? As we do this, we have the opportunity to drop in more fully with Kālī Mā, below the surface. Another layer of bliss-consciousness is waiting for us there—in fact, it is already being revealed.

With the recitation of the liturgy of the *Song of the Hundred Names of Ādyā Kālī*, we are journeying towards the center of Kālī's womb together, spiraling in and downwards into the sanctity of her dark places. This spiraling inwards is like Inanna's gates leading to the underworld where Inanna stands in front of her own dark self, her sister, and comes to terms with these aspects of herself.[14] It's not up and towards the light and somehow evolutionary. This spiraling movement is down and inward. It's not the *underworld* as this term is normally understood, however; it's the center of the yoniverse, moving towards the bindu. Our 108 nights of recitation of Kālī's hundred names is not about increasing light; it's about finding our way in the dark, towards the center, dropping into what is actually happening, not avoiding the dark or the shadow.

There is truly nothing to fear here. We are together in Kālī's lap. Moving into ourselves and her. In my own experience, moving into the dark willingly is accepting her darkness as the love that pervades the universe. It's her skin, her hair, her womb, her ways.

In order to make this passage, we will have to leave some stuff behind: old habits, beliefs, and ways of being. We enter here with our willingness to be transformed by the wisdom of the dark mother Kālī Mā. And in this, there is no up or down, nor right nor wrong. This turning towards everything with openness and allowing ourselves to transform our understandings of the dark is what allows us to fall in love—to fall in love with ourselves, our loves, and with Kālī.

She offered me an instruction on the first night of our original community recitation of the *Song of the Hundred Names of Ādyā Kālī*. The words she gave me, which I share with you here, are meant to be repeated to oneself as a reminder of what we are moving towards: "I am far more interested in you falling in love, becoming the lover, than being a decent, good, or ____ student [fill in the blank with your own habit]." Per this, and knowing how many of us are actual students enrolled in or completing programs right now, as well as how many of us are still carrying the "good student" mantle, I want to invite you to drop any notions of having to get it right, be a good student, or perfect anything. Dropping these unnecessary shells is part of the journey towards what Kālī is actually gesturing towards with her entire being. Fall in love instead, be the lover.

What would it be like to allow yourself to fall in love with Kālī, a wholehearted, messy, alive, heart-breaking, womb-opening, love affair with the divine feminine? This is such a messy and radical proposition, and it takes great courage. I know that doing this isn't easy. These 108 nights are a time of being re-made, not a time to hold it all together. "Messy" is beautiful and welcome here. It's a good thing we have each other in this, you know? We have the combined wisdom of other women and men, taking their places together, in this rich place. This convening together is itself a Yoginī Temple, old school style, for sure. In this remote open-air temple, as the nights deepen like velvet on our bare skin, what would it take for you to fall in love? Fall in love with each other and yourself and her. What would serve your body to make it a vessel available for falling in love? More baths? More anointing with rose oils? More time with the recitation of the liturgy and your shrine? This is a time for her dark love to come though, not the bright Spring love. This is the love of moon blood,[15] and the love of the dark moon. Let this be the love of making love with no lights. Can you feel what you can't see? Whatever it is, that has you more available for love and available for her darkness, please begin to do it now. Make it a part of your life during these 108 nights. We are in for a long journey and the material in this book is here to support you in this.

In this unfolding process, your shadow will surely arise to join us on this journey. Unhealed emotional and psychological wounds may be triggered. I implore you, please let this process unfold. Can you see this process as wisdom revealing itself? You will heal by bringing the wounding forth fully with kindness, love and non-judgment. Ask for support if you need it. Talk to your therapist or best friend or another yoginī or the moon or your cat. Take it all to Kālī. She is made for this. She eats it all and transforms it for us. Take it to your shrine and your practice. Her fierceness is the quality of aliveness in the midst of the dark.

I am reminded of this poem by Rāmprasād Sen, from a collection called *Grace and Mercy in Her Wild Hair*. This is Kālī Mā, indeed. Even in the pleasure and ease of her grace, beauty, and mercy, there is this ongoing thread of wild fierceness.

> Mother, incomparably arrayed
> Hair flying, stripped down,
> You battle-dance on Shiva's heart,
> A garland of heads that bounce off
> Your heavy hips, chopped-off hands
> For a belt, the bodies of infants
> For earrings, and the lips,
> The teeth like jasmine, the face
> A lotus blossomed, the laugh,
> And the dark body boiling up and out
> Like a storm cloud, and those feet
> Whose beauty is only deepened by blood.

So Prasād cries: My mind is dancing!
Can I take much more? Can I bear
An impossible beauty?
(Nathan and Seely 1999:61)

What is this impossible beauty and the related fierceness that I keep referencing? One of the Sanskrit terms often translated as *fierce* is *ugrā*.* There are many other terms but this one is often especially used in relationship to the fierce deities, the ones who dance on the shadow side like our beautiful beloved Kālī.

Ugrā is variously translated as *powerful, mighty, strong, violent, terrible, fierce, cruel, ferocious, hot* and *sharp*. Can you feel the energy resonance underneath this collection of English words? They are trying to describe something that is felt—something that is often indescribable. What is this fierce energy for? Why do we need it?

To begin in our own bodies, know that *fierceness* is the energy of the fire of transformation. Most alchemical processes require heat. The cultivation of an open body, our surrender, and the undertaking of skillful practices can generate the kind of *heat* necessary to burn off what is unnecessary. We willfully go to the fire to be transformed.

On the Tantric path, practitioners cultivate and become comfortable with all the flavors of fierceness that are in themselves, in others, in the external world, and in the deities. Most Tantric practices have been designed to actually be somewhat *confrontational*, and thus require us to have the attitude of the heroine or hero, the warrioress or warrior. Tantric practices require us to come to terms with what is unhealed, and require us to be comfortable with the dark and scary aspects of ourselves and of the world. As you might intuit by now, this Tantric worldview includes everything on the path of awakening. We leave nothing behind. In some lineages, they separate out the

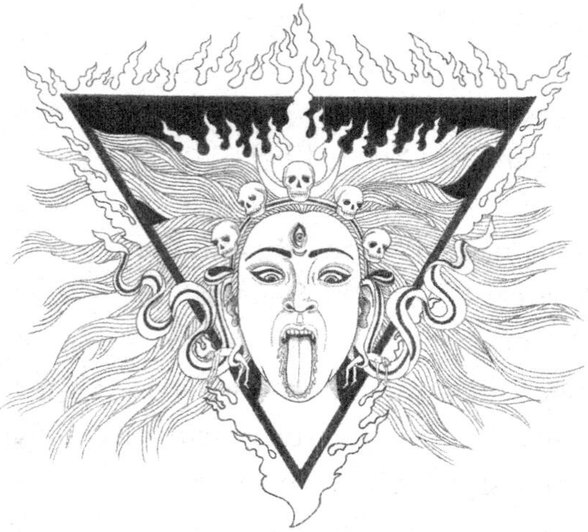

The face of transformation

challenges, perform austerities, abstain from meat, alcohol, and even from sexuality. In my lineage we might say that this form of awakening through austerities and *overcoming* is only a partial awakening because it is excluding so much.

On this Tantric path everything is included: even what I don't like, don't want, find distasteful, ugly, and painful. It is all welcome here in the lap of our Great Mother. Nothing and no one is left behind. This understanding can support us in dropping our ingrained notions of not being good enough or worthy. Our Mother Kālī not only welcomes everyone into her great lap with love, she also has the chops to eat and transform any and all of it with her great chops, her giant maw. That lolling tongue will drink it all.

Appreciating these qualities of Kālī Mā can encourage us to walk towards that which we find distasteful and painful (see the theme emerging again?). This path and our relationship with Kālī requires us at times to set down our preferences, our agendas (overt and subterranean), our boundaries, our habits, our normal ways of doing things, our controlling behaviors, our fears, and not let them limit us, neither our thoughts nor actions. We move towards what we perceive as downright unnatural, scary, ridiculous, unwarranted, distasteful, unhelpful, dangerous, and even traumatic. We walk towards it bravely, into full presencing, asking: What needs to be healed here? How do I heal it? What needs to be addressed? How can I address it? What is available for transformation? Let me transform it with her support.

Since Kālī is also the goddess of both relative and absolute time, we also have the opportunity to develop the wisdom and discernment to know when to let things take their time. Sometimes turning towards the constriction with openness isn't enough though, and we also need to work on ourselves. We may need to bring a soft sense of spaciousness, thus allowing a constriction to unfold in its own time. We allow spacious time do the healing. We can't and shouldn't force things. As a result, we begin to develop the capacity to feel into intense situations and discover what is called for, where the healing potential is, and how to move towards it with love. This requires some of that dual awareness we discussed above, that sense of being *in* the room, having our own experience, and *watching* the room at the same time. Holding this allows us to move towards all of these situations with love, grace, mercy, and tenderness—all of these are necessary even as we find ourselves dancing wildly with matted hair.

I invite you to take a minute to feel into this energy. Can you sense why undertaking the Kālī practices might be understood as a challenging spiritual path, and yet also a quick one? Sometimes it's like trying to harness a benevolent volcano without getting third-degree burns. It's no wonder that the metaphor of fire is so prevalent in Tantric deity practice: we talk of "standing in the fire," "being cooked," "standing too close to the fire," "the inner fires," "being consumed," and even the "blazing" of the inner energies. None of this is metaphoric; this is all quite literal.

Sitting with this fierce and loving goddess Kālī, in all her names and qualities, in this fierce practice of the recitation of her hundred names over 108 nights helps us to cultivate the qualities necessary to authentically move towards the realities of all existence: it's a rough and tumble world and all that we love will be destroyed sooner if not later. It goes up in smoke and flames all the time! Take care, beloveds. We cannot stave off the happenings of the world and we cannot necessarily change much that is happening. We can change how we understand what is happening, however, and build our capacity to sit with what is actually happening without smokescreens, coddling, or clinging to partial truths.

To do this, we need these fierce qualities in ourselves. The fierce deities are committed to our awakening, and I know they have to sometimes be fierce to get my attention when I've wandered off. I respond more radiantly to the slicing swords than to the coddling. That's my personality type and why this path suits me. I suspect it is the same for many of you as well. We need a kind of fierce self-determination and conviction about our spiritual journeys and what we are undertaking no matter what the outside world would say about any of this. This fierceness and intention does not override our feminine qualities but instead holds them strongly so that they are useful and useable on the spiritual path. We drop rote identities that are associated with qualities we are attached to and sit with all the flavors of experience as they arise. Our fierceness allows our opening; it supports it fully. It is not surprising that the deities in this lineage are primarily fierce. This is about potentiating fierce bliss and awareness in the yoni.

Can you feel Kālī's nourishment in her fierce blackness? The qualities of *nourishing* and *fierce* are not separate. They are cultivated simultaneously and mixed together whenever possible. Along with the application of these fierce blessings to the outer world, this cultivation process also requires us to apply them to our inner world. As Tantrikas, Kālī requires us to cultivate relentless unceasing self-love, lively nourishment, healing, surrender, a falling in love with her, a community of strong yoginīs and yogis to practice with, self-examination, and a willingness to go into uncharted territory, *mālā** and liturgy in hand.

In support of this, there are also a few qualities that we need to cultivate and utilize on the path as we begin to gather in our energies for undertaking this practice. We have to take agency and responsibility for our spiritual paths. Combined with a teacher and good companions, this will take us a long way. We have to do this work for ourselves; no one is going to do it for us. It requires fierce persistence, honesty, and capacity to keep going in the face of all we will endure on the path. We have to empower ourselves, as practitioners, with the resilience, perseverance, courage, and vitality necessary to walk this path over the long haul. And it is so worth it! The outer world will not necessarily condone us or support our spiritual practices; our fierceness and commitment to awakening in the body will take us through. This is one of the reasons why so many women who cultivate a lush interior spiritual practice do so without a lot of public notice, remaining as invisible as possible. The invisibility gives us space outside the gaze of others and allows us to follow the path as authentically as possible.

4

Śāktism, Śakti, and Tantra

Most of us have likely come into contact with the more public faces of contemporary Hinduism in the form of the gods Viṣṇu (the preserver/maintainer), Brahmā (the creator/manifester), and Śiva (the destroyer/transformer). Reverence and worship for these male deities is the focus of two of the three main tributaries of the river of contemporary Hinduism; they are sometimes referred to as Vaiṣṇavism and Śaivism, respectively. The smallest tributary of contemporary Hinduism is the one that understands goddess as primary; this branch of worship is often referred to as Śāktism. Here, the divine energies of Śakti are central to the philosophies, practices, and ways of life. Before we focus on Śāktism—the form of Hinduism where we find Kālī and her dark and fierce sisters—I want to share a little about both Vaiṣṇavism and Śaivism to give you some background.

As the name indicates, Vaiṣṇavism is the form of Hinduism in which Viṣṇu is worshipped as the supreme godhead; he is ultimate reality. Viṣṇu has wives and consorts—goddesses in their own right and worthy of independent worship—yet Viṣṇu remains the primary deity. Vaiṣṇavism is the most widespread and most public form of Hinduism. And in fact, my first contact with Hinduism, as a child, was with the Vaiṣṇavite community of Hare Krishnas in the USA. One of my mother's friends was a devotee and I remember the feasts and music with great delight.

The next largest tributary of Hinduism is known as Śaivism. There are many forms of Śaivism including both dual and non-dual lineages. Many of you might already be familiar with one of the most popular forms, which is Kashmir Śaivism, a north Indian Tantric Śaivism. Śaivism is a more inner form of Hinduism. It contains many esoteric practices, and has a heart stream that originates in Kashmir.[16] Here, devotees worship the god Śiva as the primary deity and as ultimate reality. Śiva is known for having a variety of consorts and wives, including Pārvatī and Sītā, yet none of them has the same stature as Śiva himself.

Scholars jostle about with a variety of definitions of Śāktism. My own on-the-ground experiences in Nepal and India will inform our definitions and descriptions in this book. I distinguish between two *major* forms of Śāktism in practice today, with a myriad of minor regional and cultural forms. These two major forms of contemporary Śāktism have different geographical locations in South Asia: northern Śāktism, associated with the fierce dark goddesses like Kālī, and southern Śāktism, associated with the bright auspicious goddesses such as Śrī Lalitā.[17] These northern and southern wisdom streams of Śāktism also correspond with the moon phases.[18] This is not terribly surprising, considering the cycles of the moon and our feminine flows.

The geographically southern forms of Śāktism are known as the Śrīkula[19] and revolve primarily around the Śrīvidyā lineages: the south Indian lineages of Tantric goddess worship associated with the energies and power of the full moon. Śrī Lalitā is one of the major deities and she sometimes emanates as Tripurā Sundarī or Rājarājeśvarī.[20]

The second major wisdom stream of Śāktism, and our focus in this book, is the north Indian Tantric goddess worship associated with all the forms and energies of the dark moon, known as the

Kālīkula. The Kālīkula focuses on the dark goddess Kālī and the other groups of goddesses that emanate from her and are her wisdom manifest. The goddesses include Kālī (in all her forms), the Daśa Mahāvidyā (the Ten Great Wisdoms),[21] the Mātṛkā (the Mothers),[22] and the other goddesses associated with Satī's body parts at the *Śākta Pīṭha*.*[23] The Kālīkula is geographically centered in Assam, Bihar, Orissa, West Bengal, Bangladesh, and parts of Maharashtra.

The Sanskrit term *kula** can also be understood as a spiritual family who shares teachings and practices.[24] It is sometimes also translated as "tribe," "clan," or "sacred community." Another translation of the term *kula* might be the "womb-heart gathering." The kula is the gathering of initiated devotees who share lineage, transmissions, teachings, and most especially share practices. All of these elements are understood as the "womb-heart" of Kālī or Śrī. Just as she is our womb, our heart, our heart-womb, we are hers.

These two Śākta wisdom streams, the Śrīkula and the Kālīkula, are not opposites so much as intertwined sisters, each with her own wisdoms, geographies, foci, and philosophies. Each sister has her own path, her own way, her own movements in space and time, her own flavor of womb-based śakti. Even with these differences, these sisters—Śrī and Kālī—need each other as the dark moon needs the bright moon, the night needs the day. They are in intertwined union, twins (*jami**) flowing into each other and out of each other. "This dual cosmogony represents a holistic feminine union . . ." (Thadani 1996:21).[25] Not only is there is a textual and philosophical basis for this understanding of the intertwined dual feminine nature at the basis of this worldview,[26] there is also the lived on-the-ground cultural expression. It isn't a loud or overt expression, yet for those with a subtle awareness, and infinite patience, such a yoniverse begins to make itself known.

Śāktism is a system of beliefs, practices, and sacred sites that reflect the Tantric mysteries of goddess worship with the goal of non-dual realization *in* the body, through the body, with all our sense perceptions and experiences included. These two forms of Śāktism (the Śrīkula and the Kālīkula) have a relationship to each other and to a larger yantra of practices/beliefs surrounding the body of the goddess as the entire Indic landscape.

This Kālīkula of northeast India and Nepal is yoni-heart-river-home of my relationship to Kālī. It is also among the most gynocentric spiritual lineages still being practiced today even though it is situated inside a container of culturally ingrained patriarchal worldviews and modern cultural understandings. In the northern Kālīkula, women train secretly (and without much overt acknowledgement) to cultivate a relationship with their yoni-wombs as a way to enliven relationship to Kālī, to connect with their deepest essence, to empower themselves in their spiritual endeavors, to connect with the living vitality of lineage, and to truly know themselves as divine, as the divine offering. They do this, and so do we, in order to become the love-bliss-awareness that is our true nature.

The Kālīkula is a lineage that includes the overt worship of women. As you might have intuited by now, it is not just the worship of women, there is also worship *with* women. We worship together, in community, bringing the depth of our understandings from our personal practice into relationship with our kula through sādhana. To practice with women is a vital refinement of this particular sādhana. We practice with the kula to support each other, see where we have developed, see where we need to develop, and to have role models for the path. It also creates a strong community and feeds back into our personal practices, inspiring us to more depth.

Śāktism is a vibrant wisdom stream of Hinduism, and unlike other Hindu ideologies, Śāktism tends to offer more balanced, complementary, and just forms of social organization leading some scholars to describe Śāktism, especially the Kālī worshipping forms, as "gynocentric" (cf. Saxena 2004). Indeed, the practice of Śāktism has an impact on how women understand their own spiritual practices, relationship to the divine feminine, and their social worlds. Given that women are understood as embodiments of goddess, others are able to interact with women and gain the graces of the goddess in both ritual and mundane contexts. This provides both direct and indirect support for women's empowerment, higher quality of life, and spiritual liberation.[27]

There are many different lineages within the Kālīkula, each focusing on one of Kālī's many manifestations, such as Tārā, Bagalāmukhī, or Chinnamastā-Cāmuṇḍā. While practitioners may indeed focus on the sādhanas, rituals, techniques, and mantras of a particular Devī, they are also quite at home in the temples of any of the other goddesses of the Kālīkula. For example, I have seen life-long devotees of Mā Tārā undertaking pūjā at the Kālī Mandir. Lovers of Ṣoḍaśī do not fail to bow and offer prayers to the widow goddess Dhūmāvatī, on their way to the nearby Bhairavī temple. While there may be a special deity, Devī, that each of us holds most dear, to whom we belong even, we also know that she has emanated in many forms for the benefit of all beings. To love one form of Mā is to love any of the forms of Mā. This goddess, in both her generic and specific forms, sometimes has a husband or a consort, who is also worshipped. Yet the Great Goddess is the primary focus of devotion, and ritual, and she influences everyday life in unique ways.

Given these multiple levels of complexity, it is not surprising that in Sanskrit the word *śakti* also has multiple layers of meaning that unfold in her Tantric twilight language (*sandhyā bhāṣā**). The Sanskrit root of *śakti* is *śak*, meaning "potency," "the potential to produce," "to be able," "to do," or "to act." Śakti refers to "primordial energy, the source of all divine and cosmic evolution" (Bhattacharyya 2002:139). Part of this energetic relationality is that śakti is personified in all the forms we find in the natural world.

This definition of śakti as intrinsic in the natural world around us is important as we develop our own understanding of how śakti is all-pervasive, everywhere, in everything, all the time. It is also helpful when we consider how intimately the body of the goddess, the natural landscape, and the body of the practitioner are linked.

Grammatically, śakti is a feminine noun, with feminine implications, and yet the vitality and potentiality of śakti is present in all beings, no matter the gender. Men have intrinsic śakti, as well as the ability to generate śakti through their spiritual practices, just as women do, and as all beings do. The term śakti is both a noun and a proper noun. Most generally, as a noun, śakti is the creative feminine energetic force that pervades the universe. The flavor that this energy has is *power*, and it has the nuance of being an activating power, the way that electricity has activating power. Śakti, like electricity, also has strength, and capability. Like electricity, śakti can make things happen, it creates things and also activates things. Electricity creates what is necessary for light bulbs to work, for example. Just so, śakti creates what is necessary for life to occur, for creation to light up, take form. And, as mentioned before, like electricity, śakti has the potential to destroy things.

Śakti, as a proper noun (capitalized, without italics), refers to goddess, the goddess, in her undifferentiated form, before she separates into her constituent parts. Śakti is identical to the Great Mother, Devī, Kālī, Ādyā Kālī, and is the lifeblood energy of creation.[28] She is an independent goddess, whole unto herself and simultaneously part of everything, imbued with everything.[29] "Creation is thus the self-expression of *śakti*, the subject viewing itself as object" (Bhattacharyya 2002:139). Here, as the energy arises, it develops into the polarity (or duality) that is the basis of all the forms that are this world we live in, manifest. This polarity is the basis of desire and Desire; this is Kālī's path.

All of this leads us to the next round of definitions. What is Tantra and what does it have to do with Śāktism? Śāktism is one of the types of Tantra being practiced today. I use the term Tantra to refer to the religious systems that originated in India and Nepal, which focus on the skillful devotional practices that weave the dualities into union. There are Śākta forms of Tantra, Śaivite forms of Tantra, as well as Buddhist forms of Tantra.[30] The underlying commonalities that pervade these diverse lineages and practices is that no matter the lineage or tradition, Tantra is an esoteric system in which:

> . . . dualism is an illusion, teaching that phenomenon that we may think of as opposites—like male and female, or body and mind, or divinity and devotee—are unities rather than polarities. Tantric enlightenment lies in perceiving that unity. Non-dualism is admittedly a principle taught in many branches of Indic philosophy. What makes the Tantric version of that idea distinctive is, as I understand it, its use of sexual metaphor, its emphasis upon the role of the Goddess, and its conviction that the practitioner is himself [sic] the deity (Kaimal 2002:2).

Tantric practices focus on weaving the dualities together skillfully in our body-minds through a series of skillful spiritual practices like meditation, *āsana yoga,** mantra recitation (*japa**), and a variety of secret sādhanas. Some scholars have even postulated that the root of the word Tantra means "to weave": thus Tantric practices weave together the dualities of conventional reality into the unified fabric of non-duality, or union.

Tantric practices, as they come down from the Indic religious practices, are passed on primarily orally and primarily person to person, although both scholars and practitioners acknowledge that this has changed somewhat in the past hundred years.[31] Even so, Tantra remains an *esoteric* religious system, one that has secret knowledge and practices at the core. This secret knowledge is passed on from teacher to student through the vehicle of initiation and transmission. The initiatory process—as we discussed earlier—provides the direct transference of śakti from teacher to student. Śakti is understood as the divine creative force of the universe, the divine feminine, and goddess. It is both invisible—has expression in the more-than-human realms—and can be manifested in this world as well. It can be channeled, increased, maintained, or lost in a variety of ways. The maintenance of secrecy (which concentrates śakti) is like keeping a lid on a jar of water to maintain the quality of the water. Thus, the secrecy enhances our cultivation of śakti, which we can then use to fuel our spiritual practices even further.

Śāktas understand Śāktism as the most secret of the forms of Tantric worship. There is a common saying, which I have heard in many forms: One behaves like a Vaiṣṇavite in public, a Śaivite at home, and a Śākta in secret (or in one's true heart). Another translation of this is:

> Keep your *kaula*[32] [Śākta] identity secret,
> outwardly behave like a Śaiva,
> but when in society, behave like a Vaiṣṇava.[33]

This points to how we hold these beliefs internally, in close. We train in these interior views and understandings, yet we do not disappear from the world, nor do we insist on portraying these identities in public. Instead, as part of the process of holding the teachings with care, and being in relationship with all that is, we move in the world in ways that are recognizable. We are teachers, artists, parents, friends, cashiers, computer programmers, and bakers. We live *in* the world, in union with it actually, holding this source of love in the interior mystery. I have discovered lovers of Kālī in the most interesting places as I wander in the world; they are recognizable by the light in the eyes, the playful smile on their lips under adverse circumstances, and the loving activity they offer as service to others. It's just sublime really to meet the extraordinary in the midst of the ordinary. We now know it as the expression of her grace, and all the movements of the world are her dance with Śiva.

5

The Kālīkula as Gynocentric and Womb-Centric

As we have been exploring in the previous section, the practices of Śāktism and the Kālīkula have an impact on how women understand their own spiritual practices, their relationship to the divine feminine, and to their social worlds. When fully immersed in these spiritual practices, women begin to embody a kind of spiritual discipline and inner freedom that is sublime and glorious. It is just so for men as well.

Śāktas, and other Tantrics, understand that the divine is embedded in, embodied in, practitioners' bodies, bodily experiences, minds, hearts, and emotions. As such, women are highly venerated, because there is a knowing of women as her. That said, questions emerge: How do we relate to each other from the worldview of Kālī? What is the worldview of Kālī and the Kālīkula? To address this, I want to share with you an excerpt from the *Śaktisaṃgama Tantra*.[34] This Tantra offers a glorification of the divine feminine that is embodied in living women in the Kālīkula. This understanding that all women are goddess, by mere virtue of their being in a female body, is a core tenant of this spiritual lineage. Women are venerated as goddess, and this practice offers them that realization for themselves, as well as allows relationship with others. Almost all forms of Tantric worship are based in relationality, and are meant to support the generation, establishment, and maintenance of relationships.

> Woman is the foundation of the world;
> The universe is her form.
> Woman is the foundation of the world;
> She is the true form of the body.
> Whatever form she takes,
> Whether the form of a man or a woman,
> Is the superior form.
> In woman is the form of all things,
> Of all that lives and moves in the world.
> There is no jewel rarer than a woman,
> No condition superior to that of a woman.
> There is not, nor has been, nor will be
> Any destiny to equal that of a woman.
> There is no kingdom, no wealth,
> To be compared with a woman.
> There is no prayer to equal a woman.
> There is not, nor has been, nor will be
> Any yoga to compare with a woman,
> No mystical formula nor asceticism
> To match a woman.
> There are not, nor have been, nor will be
> Any riches more valuable than woman.
> (*Śaktisaṇgama Tantra*, II.52)

This Tantric text offers us a glimpse of an embodied relational worldview that we inhabit fully for these practices to have their most beneficial and transformational effects. In our personal practices, all genders identify with Kālī: we become her in our spiritual practice, no matter our sexuality, gender, or body form. We understand that Kālī is all aspects of reality. Her hundred names can be a starting point to find our way into the illumination of this mystery.

One of Rāmprasād Sen's poems also points playfully to this Tantric mystery:

> You'll find Mother
> In any house.
> Do I dare say it in public?
> She is Bhairavī with Shiva,
> Durgā with Her children,
> Sītā with Lakshmaṇa.
> She's mother, daughter, wife, sister—
> Every woman close to you.
> What more can Rāmprasād say?
> You work the rest out from these hints.
> (Nathan and Seely 1999:55)

Beyond the worship of women, another key component of the Kālī Practices in the Kālīkula that differentiates them from many other forms of both Tantra and Śāktism is that the feminine is understood as spirit and the masculine as matter. This is a radical departure from almost every other lineage, and a radical departure from most other religious and spiritual traditions where the feminine is normally understood as matter and the masculine as spirit. Not here. This is one of the keys to unlocking our understanding of women as divine, as deity. It also helps us to make sense of many of the unique aspects of the northern Kālīkula and specifically the practice of the *Song of the Hundred Names of Ādyā Kālī* as well as other practices as they are offered here.

If we knew that every woman on the planet was Kālī (and not just symbolically, or metaphorically, or archetypically, but an actual embodiment of her), how would this change the way that we relate to each other? Can you feel into what ideas, beliefs, activities, and projections of yours would have to melt away to live into this worldview of Kālī's? Can you think of one objection, one red flag that comes up for you around this worldview? Perhaps you might work with that question over the next few days as you prepare to undertake a spiritual practice dedicated to her. Bring it forward and play with it. Examine it and see what is most real. Is there something that needs healing as a result of this examination? If so, perhaps you might consider putting out some small offerings of flowers or food for Kālī on behalf of this healing. Perhaps you might want to begin to think about creating a small shrine to Kālī and place the flowers or food there. We will go into more detail about shrines and shrine making in a little bit.

Once this understanding is established in us more, we can then begin to see all people and all existence as Kālī. We know union as a result. Can you feel this? What would it be like to not just feel this, but to know it with your entire being? What would change in your life if you truly knew this?

Those who love women have an opportunity to ask themselves an additional set of questions and engage in additional practices to support the feminine. The masculine, and all those who love the feminine, also lean into the question of how to know oneself as consort to goddess. What is it to be Śiva to her Śakti? How does one lead so she can dance us into both bliss and oblivion? What does the riverbank do to support the flowing river? How does the vine support the flower?

One of the ways that we do this is by taking up practices like mantra recitation, āsana yoga, or the recitation of the *Song of the Hundred Names of Ādyā Kālī*. We immerse ourselves in these spiritual practices so that we are able to develop our own spiritual depth and also practice in community.

The truth is that women didn't just practice with other women. Just as Śakti needs Śiva to undertake her creative work or as Śiva needs Śakti to animate, the worship of the female principle as represented by the yoni and the male principle as represented by the *liṅga** were "at the basis of a philosophical foundation of systematized Yoga" (Douglas 1971:2) and Tantra.

In Tantric practices, there is an "ideal of cooperative, mutually liberating relationships between women and men as well as encouraging a sense of reliance on women as a source of spiritual power and insight" (Gadon 2002:39 citing Shaw 1994). Women were, and are still, held in such high esteem that they were also gurus and initiators. "The high position of women in the Tantras goes against the brahmanical notion that is found in the writings of Manu" (Chitgopekar 2002:88).

> Within Tantrism then women have the authority to become priestesses and *gurus*, initiate disciples, run their own respective *asramas* and hold positions of power in the religious sphere. It is evident from the lists of the masters of several texts and from an impressive range of textual sources that many men received their first inspiration and subsequent initiation from female ascetics or Yoginis. Initiation given by a woman is considered to be more efficacious than initiation given by a man . . . . The texts claim that women are the purest source of transmission of the sacred revelation. Even to be valid as a revelation a doctrine must be revealed from the Yogini. The presence of women and women's teachings, as well as affirmations of female energy and spiritual capacities, are distinctive features of Tantric religiosity (Chitgopekar 2002:88-89).

Tantra truly celebrates, upholds, and worships women as embodiments of goddess, and as accomplished spiritual practitioners in their own right.

> Rather than degrading the female body it celebrates the sacredness of a woman's body in several forms of non-procreative yogic rituals for spiritual liberation. . . . . There is then, another viewpoint, another paradigm, of the goddess from the Tantric religion that set aside the patriarchal ethos of brahmanical religion (Chitgopekar 2002:90).

Indeed, there are also practices where women are physically worshipped as the goddess. These practices venerate young girls, married women, and even older women.

Women not only participated in these practices, but also helped to create them. As Miranda Shaw writes of the Tantric yoginīs and their circles during the early Tantric period in India: "So the women pioneered this new embodied spirituality. Their goal was to be inwardly disciplined and outwardly untamable; to be erotically alive and totally free" (Shaw 1994:148). These practices continue into the present day, influencing contemporary spiritual life. This is a gynocentric world which is distinctly feminine, engages the female energies, and is based in the body: in breath, in inhabiting the inner stillness of the heart, of yearning for union with our beloved (in whatever form that is), of fierce discipline, exaltation, devotion, and self-knowing.

6

Śakti and the Yoni as the Primordial Matrix

Perhaps you can now begin to feel something of what immersion in the Kālīkula offers us as a spiritual worldview and set of practices. Let's take these esoteric definitions and descriptions even further and begin to apply them to our own spiritual life in relationship to the Śākta Tantric practice of the *Song of the Hundred Names of Ādyā Kālī*. Questions at the heart of the recitation of this liturgy include: What is it to wake up in the body (instead of ascending out of the body)? What is it to enliven our inner worlds and relate to the deities from there? What is sacred embodiment? How do we live as the love offering that we truly are? What is devotion? What is the nature of sacred union? And what does this have to do with the Indic landscape, groups of wild and free Tantric goddesses, a menstruating goddess, and fierce desire? The exploration of these questions is at the heart of the practice of this liturgy and this book.

As a woman, in female form, the center of this divine body is the womb and the yoni, comprising the inner reproductive organs and the internal and external genitalia. Our wombs and yoni are the center of a divine microcosm of feminine energies that are the same energies that comprise all existence. Our wombs are an inner lotus that blossoms into fullness as a result of our relationship with these goddesses on our spiritual path. Underneath all this is the flow of śakti. To understand Kālī Mā, or any of the deities in this lineage of the Kālīkula, we must understand the nature of śakti and its relationship to our wombs and yonis.

In this northern form of the Kālīkula, a woman's womb-yoni is considered to be the source of the feminine energetic called śakti, the life-force energy that is the source of and animates all existence. Śakti arises out of the matrix of the womb on individual, collective, and cosmic levels. Śakti as the primordial energy of all manifest existence has three energetic forms: creation or birth, preservation, and destruction or death. All these aspects are encompassed in our inner worlds, and all are brought into our spiritual practice.

As women, in female bodies, our womb-yoni is our center and our source. This is true even for those who never had a womb or who no longer have one. It is also true for those who have never been pregnant or never had a child. The energetic system of the womb is still present even if the physical structure is not. The womb of a yoginī is the center of her body energetically, emotionally, and physically. It is her source and also the home of the divine.

The womb is where babies are created, and grown, and from where they are birthed. It is the home of our creativity, the wellspring of our vital feminine energies. The womb is the matrix from which our life force rises and to which it returns. It is the hub of our energetic and physical bodies.

The womb is also where we experience death. Our moon blood, our menstruation, is a sign that an ovum (female egg) has died without being fertilized by the sperm (male egg); it passes out of our bodies with the now unneeded uterine lining that the womb created for the possibility of growing a baby. Without fertilization, this living-nourishing matrix dies and leaves our bodies in our monthly flow (which by the way is one of the most concentrated forms of śakti in our bodies).

As such, our wombs connect us to the greater cycles of existence, including those of Kālī's primordial womb, the phases of the moon, and the oceanic tides. The cycles of birth, life, death, and rebirth are played out in our bodies in a regular cycle through the mysteries of the womb. These inner and outer mirrorings are vital components of this path. As such, in Kālī's womb, we find the sacred space to reassemble all of the parts of ourselves that we have set aside, disowned, ignored, or not fully integrated.

What might unfold for you during the recitation of the *Song of the Hundred Names of Ādyā Kālī* can bring forth wholeness and fullness on all levels and in all ways. From this perspective, you might begin to get a small sense of how the womb also has the potential to be so central to the unfolding of our spiritual paths. The cyclic nature of the womb also connects us to the womb of Devī, great goddess, so that we know ourselves as her through this homology.

Kālī is associated with the womb and the yoni. In fact, Kālī's primordial nature is associated with the womb. The Sanskrit word *yoni* has multiple layers of meaning, as is common in Tantric practices. Some of the translations include: 1. womb, vulva, vagina; 2. place of birth, source, origin, spring; 3. abode, home, lair, nest; or 4. family, race, stock, caste, etc. The word *yoni* is etymologically derived from the Sanskrit root *yuj* meaning to "join," "unite," "fasten," or "harness" (Apffel-Marglin 1987). This is the same root for the word *yoga,* which I often translate as "the art of moving into union." Thus, the yoni can be understood as that which is joining or uniting. It is active, almost an action, or activity. As women, we know that our yonis are active centers of our beings, changing moment to moment, day to day, offering us information about the state of our overall health, our internal well being, our relationship to ourselves and others. What has your yoni joined you to? In the northern Kālīkula, it links the female anatomy with the family, just as Kālī's womb/yoni links us to her in a family or kula. What are you joined to through your yoni? In the *Song of the Hundred Names of Ādyā Kālī*, there is an invitation to link our yoni to hers, to link our pelvic energies with hers, belly to belly, fire to fire.

Focusing on Kālī's yoni often reminds me of a controversial and sacred Sanskrit text called the *Yoni Tantra*. At one point, the text mentions each of the ten great wisdom goddesses, the Daśa Mahāvidyā. These ten goddesses comprise an entire *yoni-maṇḍala** unto themselves and also contain all the feminine wisdom teachings.[35] Kālī is first among these ten.[36] In the *Yoni Tantra*, each of the Mahāvidyās is associated with a different part of the outer yoni: lips, nodule, cleft, field, arch, etc.

The *Yoni Tantra* also discusses reverence for women, not symbolically, but literally. As is more and more evident now, in the Kālīkula, we revere woman *as* goddess, not *like* goddess. Doing so makes it so. I invite you, at the beginning of our practice and our offerings, to begin to come into your own knowing of the outer form of your yoni as comprised of all the forms of Kālī's yoni. Your yoni is identical with her yoni. This is enough to stop me in my tracks most days. Imagine all the lower lips as her wisdom, the hidden clitoris as her wisdom, the texture of the hair as her wisdom, the variation in color and texture as her wisdom, all the folds and forms of moisture as her wisdom. Can the most precious wisdom of the entire cosmos be found in the mystery of my yoni, your yoni, our yonis, and Kālī's yoni? I believe so. In fact, I have staked my whole life on that proposition. I am living that mystery daily. How does this feel to you? For you? Is this true for you too? I move today as Kālī's wisdom in my yoni.

What is the wisdom of our own sexual pleasure and desire in this context? What would it be like to take this knowing, or even the mental relief we might find in what I'm sharing here, and drop into our yonis and wombs, and feel/embody the knowledge that here in my body, just for today, the highest wisdoms are moving us? In fact, this wisdom stream is integral to the mysteries of the liturgy of the *Song of the Hundred Names of Ādyā Kālī*.

This worldview of the relationship between the deity and the devotee, in all parts of the body, is brought forth even more fully at the temple that is at the center of the worldview of one of the northern Kālīkula lineages. This temple in Assam is home to a yoni goddess Kāmākhyā.[37] She is understood to be inseparable from Kālī. Very simply, Kāmākhyā is the goddess of desire. *Kāma** is the Sanskrit term for "desire," and is the root word of their names, and found in the ever-popular *Kāma Sūtra*. Kāmākhyā is full blown sexual desire. What does this have to do with our spiritual path? Enlivened sexuality and the running of desire are necessary for development on this path. Please don't confuse this with much of what is labeled as "Tantra"—a set of embodied practices focused on relational intimacy and sexuality. This is not what we are talking about here. Sexual expression and the movement of sexual energy are important. Yet, it takes intense spiritual training to transform this energy from "desire" to "Desire," from "union" to "Union."

Kāmākhyā's moon flow, just like ours, is a sacred resource of śakti. Our bodies are the vessels of all the śakti we may ever need to fuel our spiritual development. Our bodies are where our depth unfoldings take place. At the Kāmākhyā temple, in the main shrine, Kāmākhyā is represented not by a statue or carving, but by a yonic cleft in the bedrock from which a spring bubbles up or pours forth. Here, we can begin to get a glimpse of how the yoni, as the heart of feminine generativity, is unified with the Kālī's wisdoms, the mysteries of her gnosis.

Kāmākhyā is herself one of the forms of Kālī, and of the goddess of desire, or kāma. In this form, she is known affectionately as Kāmākshī, or Kāmesvari (mother of love and desire, love and desire as a unified whole). One of the literal translations of her name is "Renowned Goddess of Desire" (Biernacki 2007:5). Kāmākhyā Mā sits in the center, in the bindu, of the temple hill in Assam, and also in the center of a larger cosmology revolving around the goddess' scattered body parts (which are the Śākta Pīṭha) and the Mahāvidyā.[38] Kāmākhyā takes this seat in the center of these fierce groups of goddesses because she is the primordial goddess, the yoni goddess, the premiere *yoni-pīṭha,** and also a menstruating goddess. Can you feel the śakti swirling now? It is indeed everywhere and is everything.

The most powerful manifestation of a woman's śakti is her menstrual blood. As such, here at Kāmākhyā, and for many devotees who worship śakti, menstruation is highly auspicious, potent, and full of life force, and therefore must be attended to carefully. Kāmākhyā is the *bindu** of all the Śākta Pīṭha in South Asia, around which all manifestation (and all the other body parts) swirl, ebb and flow, like great tidal forces moving and shifting in harmony with the other elemental forces.

Kāmākhyā has no form (*rūpā**) and no mūrti in which her divine presence has been installed, as is common in most other Hindu temples. Instead, she is her yoni, a cleft in the bedrock from which a spring emerges. In June, every year, Kāmākhyā and the surrounding Mahāvidyā Wisdom goddesses menstruate. It is monsoon season, and in observance and celebration of the menstruation of the goddess and the land, there is a wet, rowdy, five-day-long festival. Kāmākhyā is surrounded by the Yoginīs, the Mātṛkā, and the Mahāvidyā, just as Kālī is. Kāmākhyā is the bindu of a maṇḍala of homologies encompassing the inner and outer universes.

In the yoniverse, there are so many strong, beautiful, radiant women living into the mysteries of the womb . . . including wounding. I am aware of the women in my life who do not, in this moment, have the freedom and luxury to undergo such an exploration and spiritual practice. I am aware of the women who hold trauma in their yonis—sexual trauma, emotional trauma, and physical trauma. I am aware of the women who do not know their own sexual pleasure and the true form of freedom we embody from this form of self-knowledge. I am aware of the women all over the world whose bodies legally, socially, culturally, and ideologically belong to someone else; women are still property (overtly and subtly) all over the world. I have sobbed, moving this individual and collective wounding through my body over time.

Technically, here in the modern Western world, we are the fortunate women who have sovereignty over our bodies, although for a long time I didn't know this. I thought my body belonged to someone else. It was a long path of reclamation to truly know that this beautiful body I inhabit, no one else shall control. No one else tells me what to do with it. This is a necessary process for all of us to go through, in order to embody our own power and spiritual freedom. I'm not talking about *power over*, I'm talking about the power of being fully embodied and moving life force, śakti, through our bodies as the true offering to the divine. Moving love through this body as the divine. And this is a luxury, when we consider women's lives all over the globe.

In my lineage, we work with both the external and the internal yoni as the source of our own awakening as we unite her yoni-womb with ours through spiritual practice. And thus, we unite the life of the body, our spirit, and our sexuality. If you remember the definition of the term *yoni*, this same connection is present in the term *yoginī*. A yoginī unites all aspects of conventional reality in her body in order to "yoke" herself, join herself with ultimate reality.

In the West, there is still so much emphasis on the mastery of the body (and of sexuality) through our yogic discipline. Here, in considering the practice of the *Song of the Hundred Names of Ādyā Kālī*, we come into an awareness of another thread of the feminine yogic lineages where we unite body, mind, and spirit through body-centered practices, as well as by visualization, mantra, and spiritual practice. We awaken our own awareness, which dissolves the separation we normally feel between the internal and the external. Our suffering, according to many Tantric poems, texts, and teachings, is based in our belief that we are separate. But, goddess is always fully available to us if we can attune to her. Reciting the *Song of the Hundred Names of Ādyā Kālī* is one way that we can re-member union. Through our practices, we are able to enlarge our awareness to hold multiple realities as but flavors, or moods, of a single reality, Kālī-Brahman.

On a personal level, we cultivate a relationship with our womb and yoni as a way to deepen our relationship to spirit, to connect with our own essence, to empower ourselves in our lives, to connect with the living vitality of lineage, to discover our greatest gifts, and to truly know ourselves as divine, as the divine offering, to become the love that is our true nature. The daily recitation of the *Song of the Hundred Names of Ādyā Kālī* is an opportunity to cultivate these relationships and to engage in practices that involve coming into depth relationship with the core of our being. The relationships referred to here exist as a result of the love-stream of śakti that is the energetic breath and pulse of the universe.

We all have both aspects inside of ourselves, Śakti and Śiva, feminine and masculine. These energies play out into existence, no matter the shape, size, or form of the body, nor our gender or sexuality. These practices are about the cultivation and movement of both feminine and masculine energies, in our bodies, in order to know union. All sexes, genders, and sexualities are welcome here in the realm of Kālī, the Great Mother. No one is excluded. All are included.

Woman and the feminine energies are the embodiment of śakti (and suffused with śakti), and thus can be the activating power-source of the masculine and men, because they are the living embodiment of Bhairava/Śiva. Śakti/Kālī is in partnership with Bhairava/Śiva, the divine masculine, the godhead, all-pervading consciousness. He is the foundation, the unmoving structure, or form. His presence and reliability are the basis for all the manifestations of Śakti's dance. Bhairava/Śiva exists because Śakti/Kālī dances; Śakti/Kālī dances to enliven Bhairava/Śiva. Another way to understand it is that Śiva is the dancehall in which Kālī does the cosmic rumba, all night long, every night. So inseparable are they, that there is even a saying among Kālī worshippers in Kolkata: "'Wherever Kālī is, there is also Śiva,' (*jekhane Kālī, sekhane Śiva*)"

All we experience, and more, is Śakti's cosmic unending play and playfulness, her *līlā*,* phenomena appearing, dancing, and then disappearing. Life and death, and everything else too, are

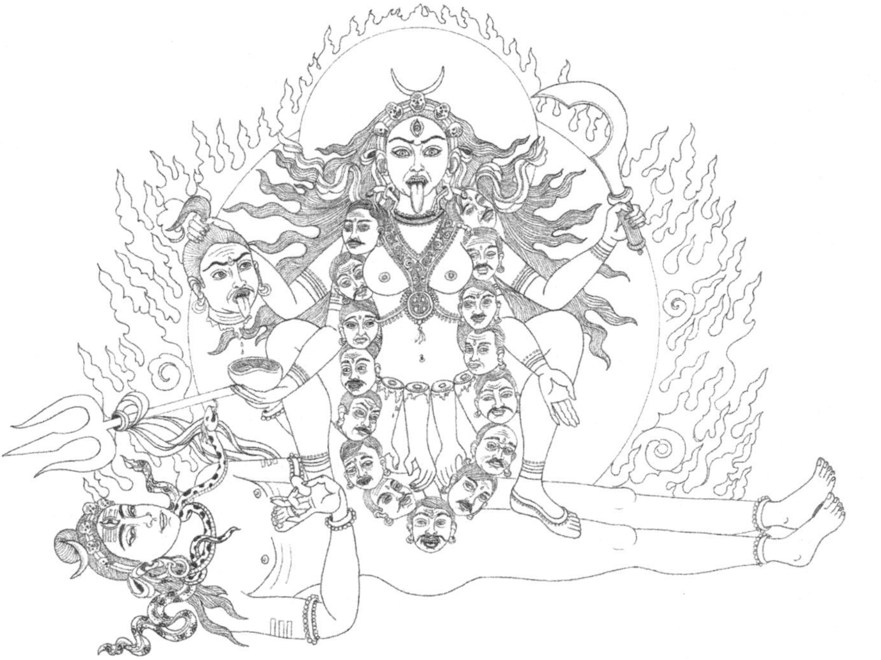

jekhane Kālī, sekhane Śiva

the expression of the mother, Kālī. Life emerges out of death as a result of Kālī's līlā, her movement, and her divine play. Death emerges out of life as well when she dances astride Śiva, stamping her ankle bells and tossing her hair. Then she dances it all to the end again, and has a smoke afterwards. She is that unruly and unpredictable.

7

Kālī's Tantras

Even though we are only part way through this Introduction to Kālī's worlds and her liturgy, the realms we are exploring are rich and intense here already. In my own experience, I've found that there isn't usually a way to move into Kālī's richness and complexity slowly and gently. With her, it's often a plunge into the vast unknown; and then we spend time coming into relationship with all that we have plunged into. So here we are floating with Kālī amidst a variety of her traditions and lineages, while all around us swirl the dynamic elements of Tantric spiritual practices and history.

This section focuses on some of the Tantric literature relevant to understanding Kālī's origins, and offers insight into the *Song of the Hundred Names of Ādyā Kālī*.

Given her complexity and the nature of Tantric paradox, it is not at all surprising to discover that there are different versions of the *Song of the Hundred Names of Ādyā Kālī*. The two most well known versions come from the *Bṛhannīla Tantra*[39] (Chapter 23) and the *Mahānirvāṇa Tantra* (Chapter 7).[40] Both versions of Kālī's names are utterly sublime in their own ways, and I highly recommend an in-depth study of both liturgies of this practice for the dedicated devotee, at some point during the 108 nights. The version we are using here, though, is based on the version found in the *Mahānirvāṇa Tantra.* One of the unique features of this version is that all of Kālī's names begin with the first consonant of the Sanskrit alphabet, *ka*.[41] This is quite stunning.

In some of the Tantric texts related to Kālī, and in the oral traditions, the Sanskrit alphabet is understood as Kālī's manifestation through sound and as sound. There is special emphasis put on the letter *ka* in the *Song of the Hundred Names of Ādyā Kālī* because this first letter is the primordial letter, the sound that is the beginning of this cycle of creation. This is the embodied resonant understanding that brings forth the matrix of primordial truth. This is the same resonant-sound-body-matrix found in this version of the *Song of the Hundred Names of Kālī*: the form of Ādyā Kālī, the primordial Kālī.

Here is another description of Ādyā Kālī from the *Mahānirvāṇa Tantra* that shows Ādyā Kālī's ways and her relationship to Mahākāla, Kāla, and Śiva, and to primordial reality as the womb-matrix.

> Thou art called Kālī because thou dost devour *Kāla*. Thou art the prime form of all. Because thou art the first in time and all elements thou art called the Prime Kālī.
>
> (After universal dissolution) assuming thy own form of shapeless darkness, beyond the range of speech and mind thou dost alone remain.
>
> Thou are with and without any form. By thy *Māyā* (illusive energy) thou dost assume many forms. Thou art the beginning of all without any beginning. Thou art the mistress of creation, destruction and preservation (Dutt 2010:100-101).

This is not a unique description of Ādyā Kālī. This understanding of her nature goes back to the first mention of Kālī (aside from the mysterious *yāmalas*[42]), which is found in an ancient Tantric scripture called the *Yonigahvara*, dating from about 1200 C.E. One translation of the title is "Recess of the Womb" (Goudriaan 1981:76). It could also be translated as "Depths of the Womb" or even "Womb Cave."[43] From the first written evidence of Kālī's nature, she is identified with the womb, the yoni.

Other fundamental elements of Kālī's ways are found in the introduction of the *Yonigahvara*: the location is a cremation ground and Bhairavī, Bhairava, and the Yoginīs are there. Bhairavī is asking Bhairava about the origins of Kālī and why she has this name. Bhairava's answer puts an emphasis on Kālī's "transcendent nature" (Goudriaan 1981:76) above all else. Here we savor another taste of the Tantric mysteries and paradoxes: Kālī's non-dual, all-encompassing, transcendent nature is anchored in the mysteries of the cremation grounds, with her usual retinue around her. Transcendent and grounded? Yes, this is Kālī's way. We come into embodiment in the intensities and harshness of the world in order that we might have access to the dance in the sky with her and her companions.

These elements are echoed throughout the Tantric literature on Kālī as well as in the practices associated with her in the northern Kālīkula. From the beginning, she is the primordial transcendent womb from which all existence arises and returns. Fierce deities, such as Bhairavī and Bhairava, worship her and Yoginīs are ever-present in Kālī's womb-matrix.

There is no single liturgy or text that structures the Kālīkula or the way the Kālī practices are lived and transmitted. In my own spiritual family, my *paramparā*,*[44] we have great familiarity with the Kālī Tantras and other left-handed Tantric texts, yet no single text dominates or guides our worldview. In addition, my paramparā picks and chooses, using some sections of some Tantras and setting aside other sections. The nature of left-handed Tantric practice is so individualized that there is no centralized instruction book. Instead, these are seen as sacred resources that we use as needed. There is so much regional variation in how Tantra is practiced, and variation from family to family, even in the same neighborhood at the same temple. The oral traditions have precedence, and then the Tantric liturgies are brought into play to support the oral traditions and practices.

8

Kālī's Names, Her Mantras, and the Nature of Transmission

Let us weave more threads of the *Song of the Hundred Names of Ādyā Kālī* together now. The liturgy of the *Song* is not a mantra, per se, yet it does have mantric qualities. As you may already know, the recitation of mantra is a powerful spiritual practice. Part of what is called forth through the commitment to a mantra practice is what is known as the "power of speech." This is what develops when we recite a mantra so completely that the shape of the sound of the mantra is inseparable from the vibratory hum of our life-force (śakti or śakti-prāṇa). When we have recited and drunk in the vibration of her mantra for so long that our body merges with her body through the vibration, this is the *accomplishment* (or the *perfection* of the power) of the mantra. This is the "power of speech." When this happens, we know that Kālī is the form of her mantra as well as the form of every one of her names.

How does this work then? In short, deities are their *bīja mantra.** The term *bīja mantra* can be translated as either "essence mantra" or "seed mantra." These powerful single syllable sounds are called "seed mantras" because they contain the entire potentiality of the deity in much the same way that a seed holds the entire potential for a tree. Thus, the mantra is the deity, in entirety. This is another one of those insights that can lead to an understanding that the Tantric path is actually not symbolic nor archetypal; it is literal. As David Gordon White writes: "much of the Tantric terminology makes sense only if it is read literally; indeed, I would argue that the ritual edifice of early Tantra only stands, that early Tantra only functions as a coherent system, if these terms are put into literal practice" (2003:8). We also have examples demonstrating this non-symbolic, or literal nature, of Śākta ritual processes from various parts of South Asia.[45] As a devotee, when I began to ingest the literalness of Tantra, I began to have the necessary interior space to allow the mysteries to unfold.

The wisdom of mantras is part of this literal Tantric mystery. When we begin to understand mantras, we also begin to discern differences among the varieties of mantras that we might be exposed to. Some mantras require transmission from the mouth of a teacher into the ear, body, and being of a student. Other mantras may be used freely, with no transmission. Bīja mantras are one of the forms of mantra that require transmission from a teacher. The topic of "transmission" is as complex as the topic of mantras. Yet, transmission is also essential to understand in the context of spiritual teachings based in lineage.

Just as there are multiple forms of mantra, there are multiple forms of transmission: there is mantra transmission, transmission to practice certain sādhanas, the transmission of lineage, and the entrustment of lineage, to name just a few.[46] The essence of transmission involves the passing of a living wisdom stream from one person to another, with a commitment/dedication/vow from the giver to the receiver and with a different but equally important commitment/vow from the receiver to the offerer.

The person who holds the wisdom stream is usually a teacher (gurvī or guru) of that wisdom stream and is deeply practiced in it. As a result, the wisdom stream of the lineage is not separate from the wisdom stream of the wisdom holder. One who has been authorized to teach can then offer a taste of this wisdom stream to another person, typically called "student," through some form of direct communication. This usually occurs orally in the case of a mantra. In most cases it is done in person even today. It is believed that the embodied presence of the teacher, in the company of a student, is most conducive to a transmission taking root and eventually coming to fruition. This direct contact is also the source for the relationality that forms the basis of Tantric spiritual practices.

My own experience of transmission is one of a river—the life-blood river of lineage that is flowing, tangible, moving, through my body, as my body fluids, in relationality. I feel it in me and it is profound, wild, real, dark red, moving mysteriously. It's being in a flow where my *sakhī*,* beloveds, kula, and deity are all immersed, and in union. They are reaching out, saying, "Come, be with us here in this love-wisdom-truth-stream."

In offering mantra and sādhana transmission to others, there is an experience of reaching out a hand, an energetic hand, and saying, "Come, join us, be with us in this living wisdom." Transmission involves a planting of a seed, an essence, in the student. The teacher asks the student: How can I help? What do you need to know this river? What embodied practices will serve your opening and movement towards your own awakening? What support am I able to be on this long complex journey?

The student, who is receiving transmission, undertakes an obligation to actively nourish and cultivate the wisdom stream that is being offered. There is also an ongoing active commitment between the teacher and the student. This mutual commitment to relationship is a form of a mystery. One of the ways this mutual commitment and mystery is played out, or enacted, is through sādhana and pūjā, the spiritual practices that include mantra accumulations and embodied union with the lineage deities.

Given all this, please know that I understand that the majority of you reading this book are not making commitments to lineage, to this kula, or to a teacher, even if you are partaking of them in this moment. This is as it should be. This book and your recitation of the *Song of the Hundred Names of Ādyā Kālī* as it is presented here are meant to offer you a dip in the river, a feast at the riverbanks, and perhaps a playful splashing with friends.

Having explored the many aspects of transmission, we move now to consider the power of mantra. What is the power of mantra, then? When linked with the power of transmission, and coming from a commitment to a sādhana (including intensive mantra practice or the recitation of the *Song of the Hundred Names of Ādyā Kālī*), Kāmākhyā-Kālī takes our hand and shows us how to cultivate our ordinary relationship with desire and transform it into a sacred relationship with desire. The desire that is śakti has the power to move us into more profound embodied awakening on our spiritual paths, and this is what I sometimes call "union."

> Kālī is the beginning, the bindu of creation manifest as desire, kāma, the creative essence of the cosmos.[47]

To practice into union in the Kālīkula, there is a special emphasis on mantra recitation. Again, it is the way to link ourselves to Kālī, in all her forms, and creates a radically new way of relating to others. More specifically, mantra practice eventually allows us to enter into other sādhanas of this lineage.

As mentioned, the recitation of the *Song of the Hundred Names of Ādyā Kālī* is not a mantra practice in the most formal sense. Yet, there are enough mantric elements here including the use of seed syllables, the opportunity to drop into devotion, and how the sound vibration of the recitation of the names, like with a bīja mantra, allows the worshipper to unite with the deities. This is what I call the "yoga of union."

A bīja mantra is comprised of single seed syllables based on the letters of the Sanskrit alphabet. Combined with other words and additional bīja, bīja mantras are the main form of mantra used during the spiritual practice of japa, where we repeat a single mantra over and over again, usually with a rosary (mālā). According to one Tantric interpretation, the tattvas (or elements, as you may recall) not only unfold through light, but also through the recitation of the letters of the alphabet: sound is the pathway that allows light to pass into form. The letters are not mere sounds denoting specific meaning, but are powerful enough to create, preserve or destroy the cosmic system (Aryan 1980:9). The garland of the letters of the Sanskrit alphabet, the *varṇa mālā,** are the basis for the Tantric bīja mantra and constitute the efficacy of the mantra itself. Every vowel and consonant has a primary meaning that arose out of this essential primordial śakti. This is relevant here because the *Song of the Hundred Names of Ādyā Kālī* begins with three bīja mantras connected to the first three names in the liturgy: *hrīṃ*, *śrīṃ*, and *krīṃ*.[48]

Beyond the bīja mantras, there are other categories of mantras such as gāyatrī mantras. In the West, many of us are familiar with what is known as the Gāyatrī Mantra. In truth though, there is not a single Gāyatrī Mantra: there are many many gāyatrī mantras. Each deity has their own gāyatrī mantra, which is a traditional meditative aid. We use gāyatrīs to pray for the presence of our personal deity (*iṣṭadevī* or iṣṭadevatā**). Gāyatrīs are usually twenty-four syllables long.

The other form of a mantra with which you may have some contact is the *praṇām mantra*:* these are longer mantras that usually end with the words *svāhā* or *namaḥ*. A praṇam mantra offers homage, praise, and supplication to the deity.

If yoga is the art of moving into union, then mantra recitation is one of the yogas (tools, practices) that we use to bring our body/mind/spirit into union with the deity, irrevocably. Perhaps you can now begin to feel the potency of starting a recitation such as this with the power of bīja mantras?

The first three names of the *Song of the Hundred Names of Ādyā Kālī* incorporate these same qualities in the connected bījas: *hrīṃ* is the sound of generation, *śrīṃ* is the sound of preservation, and *krīṃ* is the bīja of transformation.[49] Along with the power of these bījas embedded in both its beginning and end, the entire *Song* is also considered a kind of mantra, and each of her names is also a mantra. The recitation of the entire *Song* is the utterance of mantra embedded in mantra, and again embedded in mantra. This nested and multilayered rendering of mantra is powerful, and when done over time, and with devotion, can begin to reveal some of the depths of Kālī's mysteries.

With all of this background material, now, let us move into a more concrete conversation about how you might begin this spiritual practice—focusing on the recitation of the *Song of the Hundred Names of Ādyā Kālī*.

9

How to Practice the Song of the Hundred Names of Ādyā Kālī

We have been talking about undertaking the *Song of the Hundred Names of Ādyā Kālī* as a spiritual practice. What does this mean? One sublime rendering of the meaning and usefulness of spiritual practice that was offered to me by a beloved is that a spiritual practice, such as the recitation of the *Song*, is the *enactment* of the deity. Another way of saying this is that our spiritual practice allows us to be "one with thee."

A spiritual practice is an ancient embodied technique that offers us the opportunity to fall in love with the deity, with Kālī. We undertake a spiritual practice like the *Song of the Hundred Names of Ādyā Kālī* because it is the foundation for the long-term love affair with her. I remember when I first began to learn the formal structure of a Kālī practice inside my spiritual family in Assam, India. Before this, I had a more freeform love affair with Kālī that followed my own moods, whims, and desires. After some time in this self-directed mode, I was no longer making progress in my relationship with Kālī and I actually felt that I was backsliding. I had enough experience to know that it was time to find a qualified teacher to help me move more profoundly (and precisely) into my relationship with Kālī and a spiritual path. I was hungry for more, and discovered that my own self-direction could only take me so far.

I undertook a long journey that eventually led me to meet my spiritual family at the temple for the goddess Kāmākhyā in Assam, India. And, having arrived among them, and once basic formalities were made, they insisted, despite all the education I had, and research I had undertaken, that I sit in formal practice in the small family temple dedicated to the Mahāvidyā Bhairavī near Kāmākhyā's main temple. I felt stifled and controlled by their instructions: to sit in front of the shrine, with nothing but a small burlap sack under my hips for cushion, and undertake a strict and formal mantra practice. Really? This was useful? Repeat this simple mantra over and over?

I was quickly quite bored by the whole thing. I thought I was above this, beyond this, too good for this. My body ached from sitting relatively motionless on a hard concrete floor. It was far too hot to relax. I wanted to be outside wandering around, drinking chai, talking to people, and doing my own thing.

But there was Mā, inside the temple looking back at me. Offerings were set out and flower garlands were draped around her. Other devotees would wander in and out paying obeisance. I tried to let myself drop into the rhythms of sitting with nothing to do but recite a mantra and keep track of how many times I had recited it. I rejoiced when we got up to relieve ourselves outside or go back to the house for a meal. I hunkered down and pouted inwardly as we made our way back to the temple for the next session. Where was my joy? What had happened to my personal self-directed love affair with Kālī? I was sullen and disappointed. In the process, somehow, my resistances and patterns were slowly worn down; I began to feel small moments of joy. I found that the more I surrendered, the easier it was. My fighting was what made this hard. My presumptions about what spiritual practice looked and felt like were what was causing my suffering. My discomfort was the result of my own habits and beliefs.

Days continued to pass, turning into weeks; a routine developed. I found myself dropping into her lap more and more as I recited the mantra and went into this new and uncomfortable process. I knew from all my academic research, and from my time in Kathmandu, that formal mantra practice was an ancient Tantric technique, highly valued among all the practitioners I had met or read about. And, in truth, in other contexts, I loved reciting Kālī's mantras. I knew that there was wisdom for me in this; I just hadn't had much experience going into this ancient wisdom for myself. To *have* to sit there and do this just because they said it was good for me? Goddess, I felt like a rebellious teenager, and I imagine that from my family's point of view I was.

Besides my own love of Kālī, the other piece that was extremely supportive was that I was fortunate to have good company practicing with me, both on my right and left sides. I was not alone. These spiritual companions helped get me into my seat (āsana) each day, kept me in my seat during the long practice sessions, helped me begin to feel what it would be like to willingly "take my seat" in the midst of the strains of hour after hour of japa. I rebelled. I cried. I glowered. I argued. Why did I have to do *this*? What good was this when I already had a love affair with Kālī? Yet, my companions loved me enough to persuade me to stay put and keep going. Hour after hour, day after day. Days stretched into weeks, and yes even further into months. We kept going. I kept going. I surrendered in small increments. I allowed myself to feel their love for me, and I allowed myself to soften into their love and let the practice wash through me. At some point, I stopped fighting. I just relaxed and opened. I kept going. We kept going. I discovered something in this process that I hadn't had access to on my own. Some of the discoveries were subtle, like how to become more comfortable sitting on a concrete floor over the long haul. Or how my subtle body opened in the presence of jasmine flower garlands. Or how the soft hum of mantra vibrated my being in ways that were exquisitely pleasurable. Or how my breath and the breath of my companions had synced. Or how we moved as one instead of separately. Other changes were more overt, and still other effects only blossomed into full-blown transformations a long time later. I remember one profound day, half way across the world in the middle of teaching a classroom full of college students, the potency of those spiritual practices filled me as I wrote on the white board. I was dizzy with the fragrance of it.

Over time, I fell in love with Kālī in more profound ways that I didn't know were possible. I discovered the wisdom of the ancient ways. I settled in and let myself go. I learned to trust these people and the practice and the endless recitation of her mantra.

My hope for you is that your own intuition and yearning will support you in beginning to learn to trust this practice of the *Song of the Hundred Names of Ādyā Kālī* in much the same way. As I hope this sharing illustrates, undertaking a regular and disciplined spiritual practice is one of the most reliable ways for the fruit of all this to develop, and for the energies to penetrate the cells of our bodies, transform our minds, and affect our lives.

Our beginning, then, is the profound opening you may already have towards implementing a regular spiritual practice to embrace your relationship with Kālī. You have come this far in the book, and I wonder if you can feel some soft place in you that desires a richer and more vibrant connection with Kālī? Can you feel your own desire for union with her? If so, can you feel into this desire a little more and find the place where you might consider committing to a spiritual practice for the sake of quenching this thirst for union with Kālī? Can you find a place in yourself that is open to the development of a more profound and nourishing relationship with Kālī through the recitation of the *Song of the Hundred Names of Ādyā Kālī*? If so, this is your starting point. This is the beginning. Welcome.

One of the most fruitful ways to proceed is to consider reciting the *Song* every night for a set period of time. Perhaps begin with a commitment of a week. Or perhaps make a commitment that runs from one dark moon to the next dark moon? A traditional period of time for a commitment like this is 108 nights. Perhaps try out a shorter time span first and see how you feel. You can build towards the fuller 108-night commitment over time.

Our daily practice and our commitment to developing a relationship with Kālī are two of the most reliable things in our lives. No matter what else is happening, no matter world circumstances or personal situation, sādhana and my relationship with Kālī is stable and foundational. I exhale because I have this foundation; and no one gave it to me even though others gave me these practices. I gave myself this gift of love, support, nurturing, nourishing, healing, depth, and union by coming to my practice regularly, steadily, over time, no matter the circumstances.

Once you have decided on the length of your practice commitment and the starting night, it is time to consider what this nightly practice might look like. An entire recitation of the *Song* (with both the Sanskrit and the English) takes about twenty to twenty-five minutes.

I recommend that you recite the liturgy speaking aloud both the Sanskrit name and English translation. Use the names with the numbers in front of them for this. For example, I would recite the first two stanzas like this:

> *Hrīṃ* Kālī; *Śrīṃ* Karālī (She Who Is Formidable, Dreadful), and *Krīṃ* Kalyāṇī (She Who Is the Bestower of Wellbeing). Kalāvatī (She Who Is the Possessor of the [64] Arts); Kamalā (She Who Is the Lotus); Kalidarpaghnī (She Who Destroys

> Pride during the Kālī Yuga); Kapardīśakṛpānvitā (She Who Gives Grace to the One of Matted Hair); Kālikā (She Who Is the Devourer of Time); Kālamātā (She Who Is Mother of Time) and Kālānalasamadyutiḥ (She Who Is as Radiant as the Fires that Consume the Universe); Kapardinī (She Who Has Matted Hair) Karālāsyā (She Who Has Fangs and a Formidable Expression) Karuṇāmṛtasāgarā (yet also She Who Is the Oceanic Nectar of Compassion).

A nightly recitation would include the full list of her names as well as the reading of one of the contemplations. Start at the beginning of the Contemplations, reading one per night, in the order that they are given. Don't skip around in the Contemplations. They make the most sense in the order they are offered, as the names build on each other as you do the recitations. If you are doing a weeklong practice commitment, you would read the first seven names in order, night by night. If you are doing a month-long practice commitment, you would read one contemplation daily for thirty or thirty-one days. Once you have completed your practice commitment, you may feel moved to begin a second commitment for a longer period of time. Under these circumstances, you would start all over again at the beginning of the Contemplations. The generation of the flow of the names and the contemplations, from beginning to end in order, is part of the mystery of this spiritual practice, as well as part of the unfolding of your relationship with Kālī.

In the beginning, I also recommend that you undertake the recitation of the liturgy out loud to support your experience of generating the sounds and words, and of having them move through your body into the world. This is a vital part of the practice. By reciting it out loud, you are activating the mantric properties of the *Song* as well as taking your practice into your own hands and making it your own. This is the way that your personal relationship with Kālī will develop. Having her names in your mouth and on your lips is the greatest source of connection and depth in this spiritual practice.

If you do this for awhile, you will find yourself dropping into the flow and rhythm of the liturgy with resonance and connection. After some time, you will have enough familiarity with the meaning of the names to be able to undertake the recitation of the names in Sanskrit only. To begin though, I recommend using both the Sanskrit and the English for the names so that you begin to have familiarity with the meaning along with the blessings of the Sanskrit sounds.

In this Tantric liturgy of the *Song of the Hundred Names of Ādyā Kālī*, we are focusing on the dark goddess Kālī in her primordial form as Ādyā Kālī. In this context, we have the opportunity to move into lush embodied states with Kālī as our Beloved. I would go so far as to say that we do spiritual practice because it serves as a vessel, a container, a matrix within which we meet our love affair with Kālī. From this perspective, we can realize how spiritual practice is the *remembrance of union with Kālī.*

Now that you have familiarized yourself with the liturgy and have contemplated a commitment to recite the *Song* for a set number of days, it is time to establish a shrine to her. This is part of the necessary preparation for undertaking a practice commitment. This shrine should be devoted to Ādyā Kālī alone and the recitation of her hundred names. This is not to disrespect or disregard the other deities that you may have relationships with. I encourage you to keep your other altars up, if you have them. What I am pointing to is the importance of a dedicated altar for the practice of the *Song of the Hundred Names of Ādyā Kālī*. The singularity of your Kālī shrine will support you in discerning the specific energies that Mā Kālī offers, as well as in developing an undistracted relationship with her. Here is where your relationship with her will take root and flourish. This shrine is also a strong support for your personal practice and for your practice commitments; it offers a rich foundation.

To set up this shrine: Find an image of Kālī that appeals to you, or perhaps you have a statue already. Make this the centerpoint of the shrine. If you have a red or black scarf or piece of material, you can use this as the altar cloth.

If you have used a "womb pot" on your shrine before, please install it anew on the first day of your recitation of the *Song of the Hundred Names of Ādyā Kālī*. For those who are new to this aspect of a Tantric shrine, the womb pot (also called a *kalaśa*, or *ghaṭa*) is the womb/crucible/container of Ādyā Kālī in living embodied presence. She lives on your own shrine, in your home, and thus her home is there too, with you. Having a womb pot on the shrine is an honoring of both Kālī and yourself as a devotee. In terms of shape and size, these pots are generally rounded with a narrower neck and a wide mouth. If you don't have something like this already, you might consider buying a small traditional one. One of the other terms for this vessel (before it is consecrated) is *lota*, and I've seen them on eBay under this search term. You might also be able to find them at Indian markets if you live in an urban area. My womb pot is on the smaller size (compared to what I've see at temples in India) because I often travel with mine. It's much

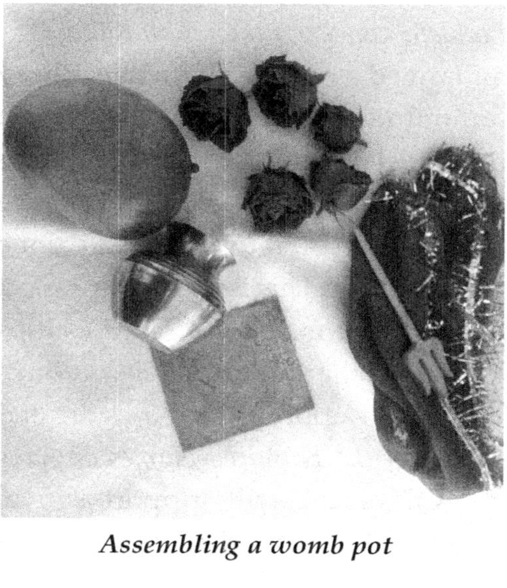

Assembling a womb pot

easier to travel with smaller ritual items than larger ones. I also like one that a small pomegranate or apple can sit on top of comfortably. With an appreciation for your responsibilities and your lifestyle, as well as the size of your shrine, decide what works for you. You can be innovative with this too, noting what works in terms of your relationship with Kālī.

The womb pot/yoni crucible on your shrine should be in a central position. To do this, first clean the pot well, letting it dry. Put a couple of grains of rice or flower petals on the spot on the shrine where the pot will live. If you have one, you may use a small paper or copper Kālī yantra instead of the rice or petals as the seat for the womb pot.[50] Set the pot on the flower petals, rice, or yantra. Fill the pot just to the neck with clean water. As this is a Tantric practice, you may want to add a couple of drops of wine or whiskey, or other strong alcoholic beverage. This should come from an unopened bottle, reserved for offerings to Kālī.

We will use the *yoni-mudrā** to activate Kālī's womb pot. A mudrā is a physical gesture used in ritual contexts that invokes and moves specific energies for specific purposes, normally inside of a sādhana or other ritual practice. Sometimes the term *mudrā* is translated as "seal" pointing to how a mudrā can be used to "seal" energy into a particular place or form. Mudrās are a tangible way of bringing energies into form, and a way to enhance our embodiment of those energies. An example of a mudrā that many of us may be familiar with is to bring our hands to the center of our chest in prayer position, this is technically called *añjali mudrā*.* It is the gesture of the lotus beginning to bud, and is often used in greeting. This mudrā, as the lotus unfolding,

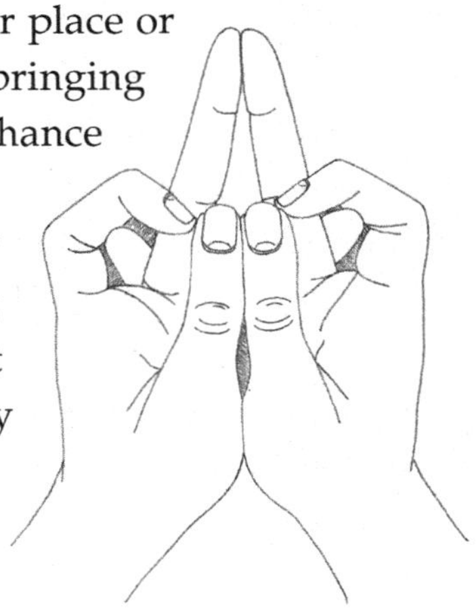

A version of the yoni-mudrā

gestures towards the awakened state that is inherent in each of us. When we embody this mudrā, the mudrā invokes the state, is a remembrance of the state, and is the state itself, all inseparably. There are countless mudrās in the ritual lexicon, and often several variations of each mudrā, depending on the tradition or lineage, and on the level of initiation (complexity tends to arise with different levels of initiation). In addition, our entire body can be understood as a mudrā, a gesture of our innate awakened nature. From this perspective, sometimes in the world of secret Tantric ritual and twilight language, mudrā is one of the terms that might be used to refer to a female practitioner.

Now, formulate an intention to activate her womb pot and offer the yoni mudrā over the mouth of the womb pot while reciting Kālī's bīja mantra three times. Articulate your intention for her to come and reside here on your shrine. The womb pot will now be activated: this is Kālī's living womb. Treat her with care and devotion.

At this point, you may anoint her womb pot with a little sandalwood paste or *sindūr** if you'd like, marking her body. Technically, Kālī is naked at this point. If you have a small piece of beautiful cloth, you can dress the womb pot in the cloth by wrapping it around, in a lovely way, as though putting on a sari. Place five green leaves around the neck of the womb pot (mango leaves are traditional for this), and place a small piece of fruit, such as an apple or pomegranate, on top of that. This piece of fruit is Kālī's head. I sometimes use a flower for this, such as a hibiscus or large rose, if I can't find an appropriately sized fruit. Your womb pot will remain on the shrine for the entire length of your practice commitment (whether a week, a month, or the entire 108 nights). This is Kālī, incarnate, in your home.

You can also offer other adornment to the forms of Kālī on your shrine including the womb pot, such as mirrors, eyeliner, henna powder, or any form of adornment you think she might enjoy. She especially loves red. It is best to offer her new things, not leftovers or partially used items. If you don't have these things, it's fine. Your own heart's devotion is the true offering, and you can begin to build towards this during this practice.

On the first night of your recitation of the *Song of the Hundred Names of Ādyā Kālī*, please have a small set of offerings ready for the shrine that include the five *makāra*:* meat, fish, wine/alcohol, some puffed grain (mini rice cakes will work), and some offering that represents union to you.

What I am describing as "union" here is actually called by the term "mudrā" in the Tantric literature and in Tantric culture. Here we see how, as noted earlier, that mudrā can be multivalent. Mudrā refers to a female practitioner of some Tantric rituals as well as to the grain offering. What is at stake here is that any mudrā, no matter the form, is an embodied gesture towards awakening or union. This is a side note, but a rich one: in much of the Tantric literature and culture, it is common to use Tantric "twilight language" (sandhyā bhāṣā), the coded language used to conceal the inner meanings from the uninitiated or outsiders. It is understood that each term, or description, in Tantra can have multiple levels of meaning that are unveiled to the practitioner over time either as a result of direct experience or as a result of instructions from the heart-womb teacher (gurvī or guru). Some of the most esoteric aspects of Tantra were concealed and protected, in this way, so that the lineage stream might continue to flow no matter whether the external cultural conditions were hospitable. This many-layered meaning found in Tantric language is also a teaching on how richness of experience emerges over time and with ongoing contact. What we first see on the surface is not the depths. In addition, our own experience and spiritual depth will ripen over time. Tantra's use of twilight language points to this as well. The offering of the five makāra has multiple layers of meaning that will unveil themselves through study, practice, contemplation, and through your own direct experience. As you shop and prepare the food, ask yourself what is below the surface activity? What ancient wisdom is at play here? What do the five makāra convey? What is Kālī's relationship to them? What is yours? Feel into all of this and let it unfold over time; there is no hurry here.

Now that we sense how the Tantric makāra offerings might have multiple levels of rich unfolding meaning, it is time to arrange these offerings for the shrine. Place some of the offerings on a single plate for Kālī and her consort. You might want to put the heads of flowers on the plate as well, or other gorgeous decorations. You can place this plate either on the shrine or in front of the shrine. At times, I have used small folding tables or trays for this purpose so that the offerings are off the floor and at about the same height as the shrine. You can also make plates for yourself, your teachers, and any others participating in the ritual. Pour the alcohol offerings as well.

You may feel moved to make a moon blood offering to Kālī. If so, now is the time to place a small bowl of moon blood on the shrine. For men, or for those of us who are holding our blood inside, a small bowl of red wine is a good substitute offering.

Fresh flowers are so beautiful for the shrine. The tops of flowers can be placed around the shrine to decorate and bless your offerings. I often make small garlands of flowers out of mini red rose buds for the Kālī statues on my shrine. I also like flowers in a vase to heighten the beauty, sensuality, and sacredness of the space. Clearly, something special is happening! Kālī especially loves hibiscus flowers and jasmine. Yet any red or fragrant flower will do.

Now, with a familiarity with the liturgy, the components for a practice commitment, and the makings of a shrine, begin to consider what you would like to dedicate your practice to? Is there an energy you would like to cultivate, or a healing or insight that you need? Perhaps you just want to fall in love? Whatever it is, consider journaling about this, and including some representation of this on your shrine. Feel the fullness of the potential in all of this. Feel her love permeating all of this.

May we be protected, may we be healed, may we be whole, and may we know our own selves. May our innate wisdom as women and men manifest. May we wake up in these bodies, in this lifetime, in the same maṇḍala. I dedicate my practice during this sādhana to the healing of the wombs and yonis and lives of women everywhere, and to our awakening as embodied yoginīs and yogis. May it please you, may it please her, that we share this sādhana together.

II.
SONG OF THE HUNDRED NAMES OF ĀDYĀ KĀLĪ

आद्याकालिकादेव्याः शतनामस्तोत्रम्

ādyā kālikādevyāḥ śatanāma stotram
Song of the Hundred Names of Ādyā Kālī

(also known as *ādyākālī svarūpa stotram* and as the *Tantrik Hymn to Kālī*) from traditional tantric textual and oral sources of the *Kālīkula*

I remember again and again the dark primeval Devī swayed with passion.
Her beauteous face heated and moist with the sweat [of amorous play],
Bearing a necklace of Ganjā berries,[1] and clad with leaves.
Tantrasāra 15 (Avalon 1964:35)

ह्रीं काली श्रीं कराली च क्रीं कल्याणी कलावती ।
कमला कलिदर्पघ्नी कपर्दीशकृपान्विता ॥

hrīṃ kālī śrīṃ karālī ca krīṃ kalyāṇī kalāvatī |
kamalā kalidarpaghnī kapardīśakṛpānvitā | |

1) *Hrīṃ* Kālī
2) *Śrīṃ* Karālī (She Who Is Formidable, Dreadful), and
3) *Krīṃ* Kalyāṇī (She Who Is the Bestower of Wellbeing),
4) Kalāvatī (She Who Is the Possessor of the [64] Arts),
5) Kamalā (She Who Is the Lotus),
6) Kalidarpaghnī (She Who Destroys Pride during the Kālī Yuga),
7) Kapardīśakṛpānvitā (She Who Gives Grace to the One of Matted Hair),

कालिका कालमाता च कालानलसमद्युतिः ।
कपर्दिनी करालास्या करुणामृतसागरा ॥

kālikā kālamātā ca kālānalasamadyutiḥ |
kapardinī karālāsyā karuṇāmṛtasāgarā | |

8) Kālikā (She Who Is the Devourer of Time),
9) Kālamātā (She Who Is Mother of Time), and
10) Kālānalasamadyutiḥ (She Who Is as Radiant as the Fires that Consume the Universe),
11) Kapardinī (She Who Has Matted Hair),
12) Karālāsyā (She Who Has Fangs and a Formidable Expression),
13) Karuṇāmṛtasāgarā (yet also She Who Is the Oceanic Nectar of Compassion),

कृपामयी कृपाधारा कृपापारा कृपागमा ।
कृशानुः कपिला कृष्णा कृष्णानन्दविवर्द्धिनी ॥

kṛpāmayī kṛpādhārā kṛpāpārā kṛpāgamā |
kṛśānuḥ kapilā kṛṣṇā kṛṣṇānandavivarddhinī | |

14) Kṛpāmayī (She Who Is Full of Grace),
15) Kṛpādhārā (She Who Is the Vessel of Mercy, the Supporter of Grace),
16) Kṛpāpārā (She Whose Mercy Is Without Limit, She Who Is Beyond Grace),
17) Kṛpāgamā (She Who Is Attainable Only by Her Mercy, She Who Moves in Grace),
18) Kṛśānuḥ (She Who Is Fire, the Female Deity of Fire),
19) Kapilā (She Who Is the Tawny-Colored One),
20) Kṛṣṇā (She Who Is Black),
21) Kṛṣṇānandavivarddhinī (She Who Is the Increaser of the Bliss of the Dark One, Kṛṣṇa),

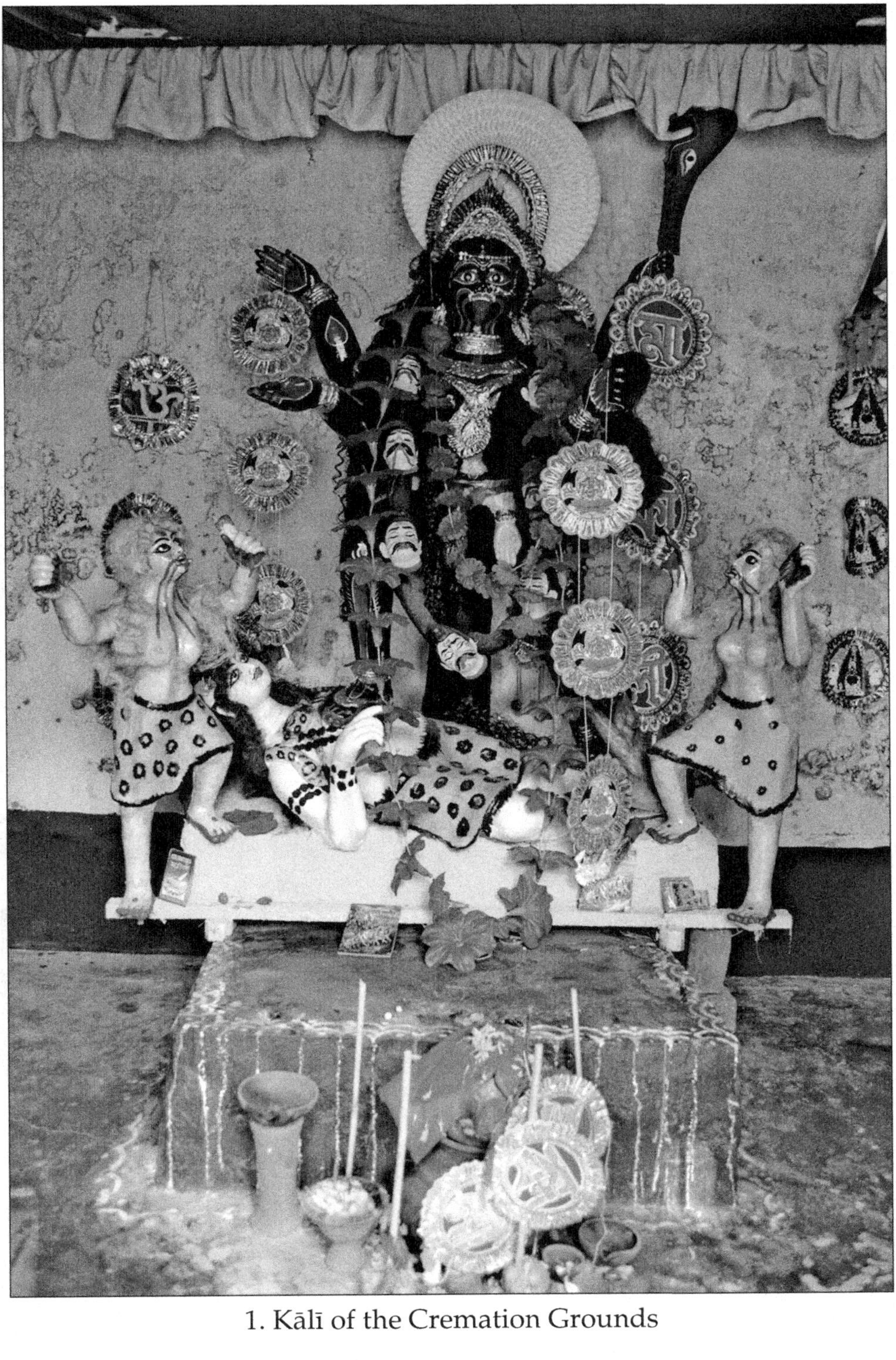

1. Kālī of the Cremation Grounds

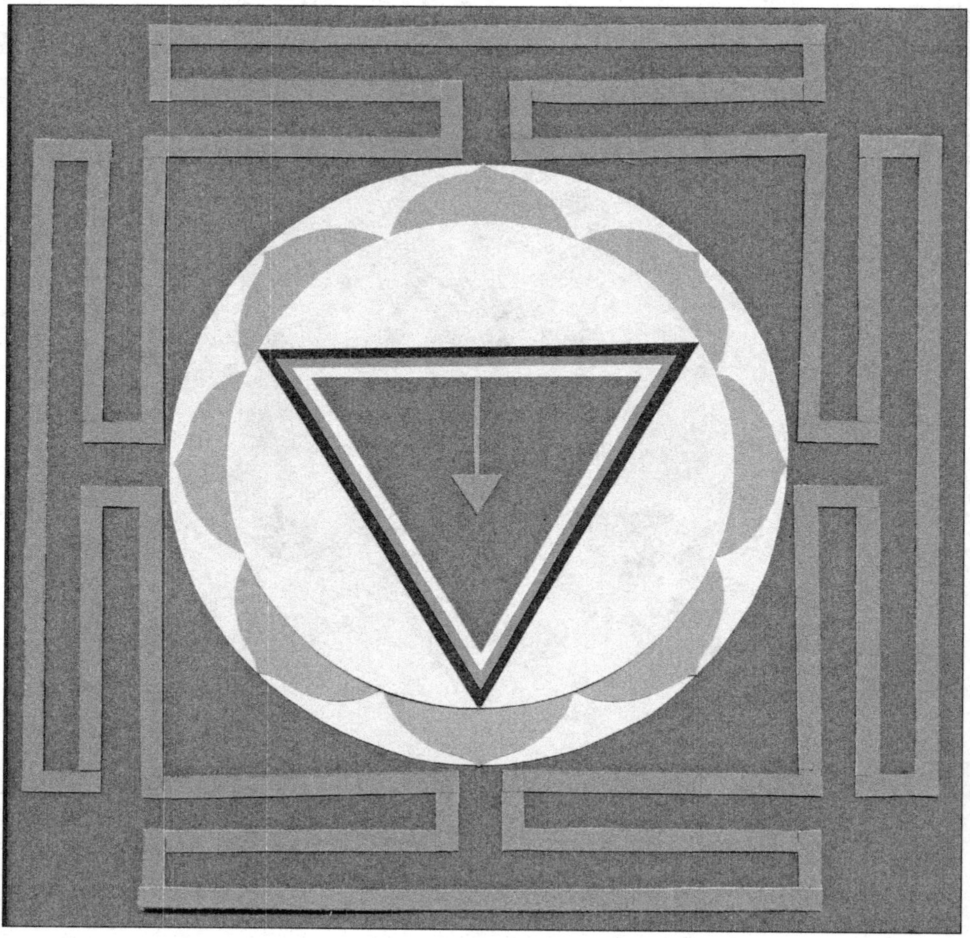

2. Kālī Yoni Yantra

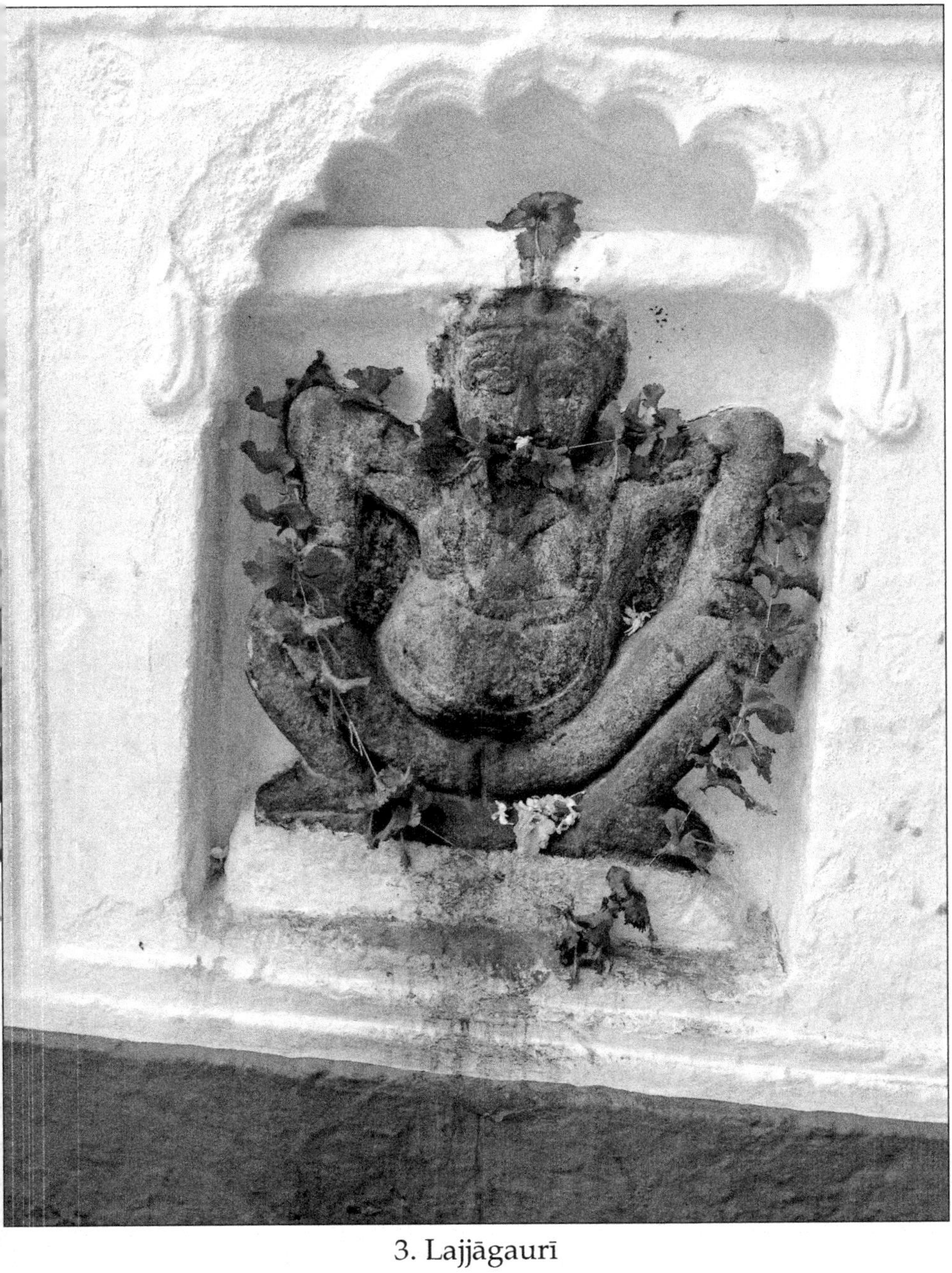

3. Lajjāgaurī

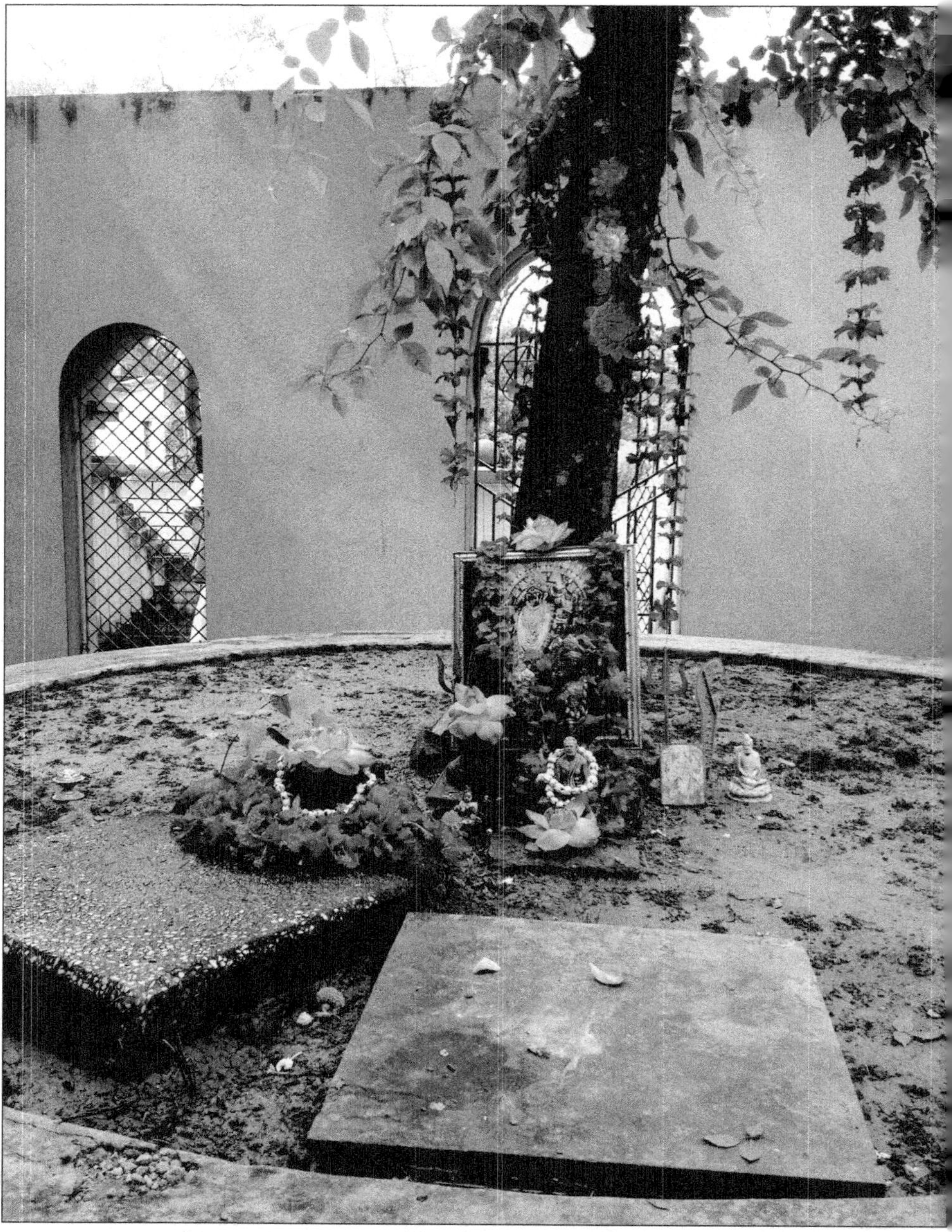

4. Shrine to Bhairavī Brāmaṇī (aka Yogesvarī)

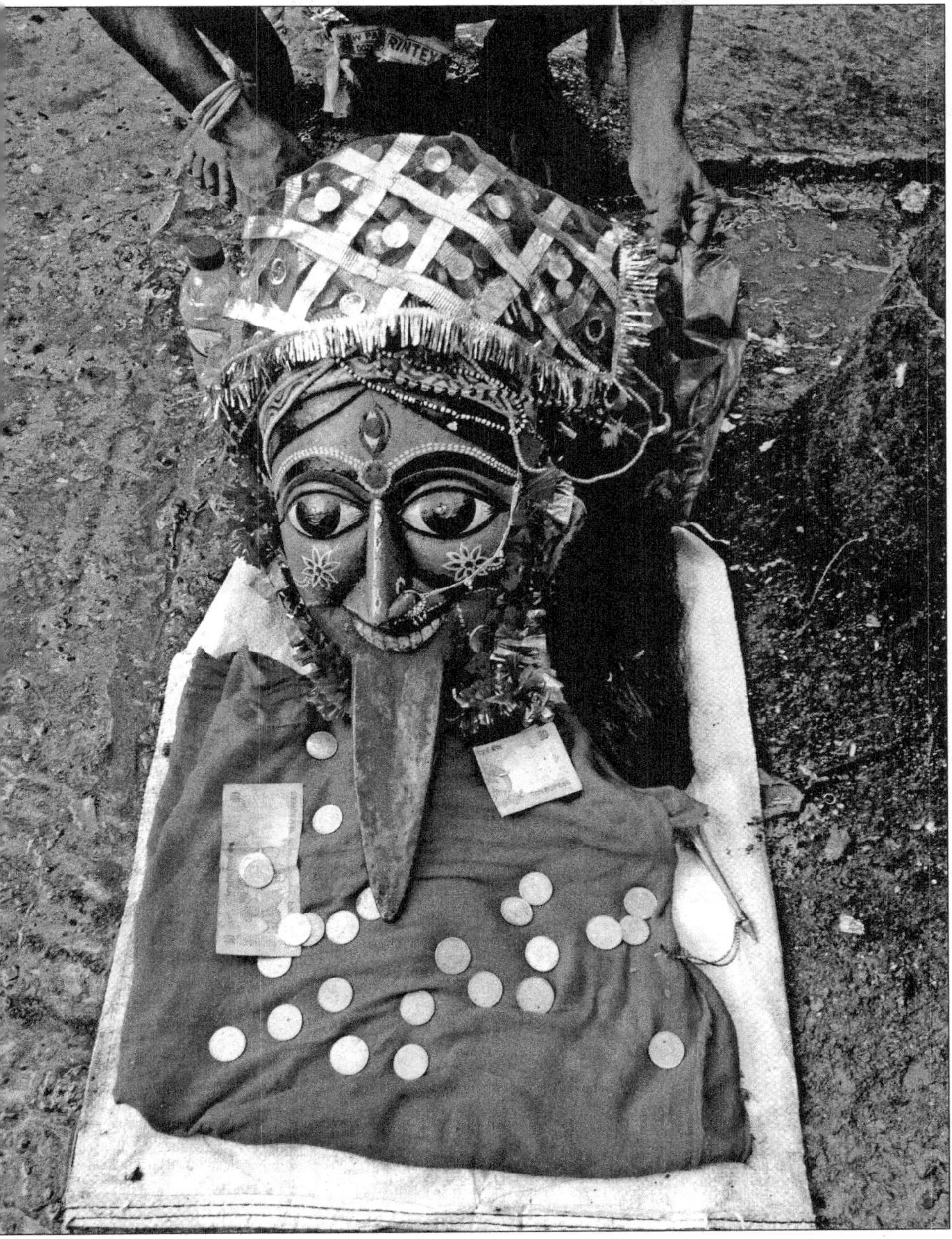

5. Kālī's Tongue

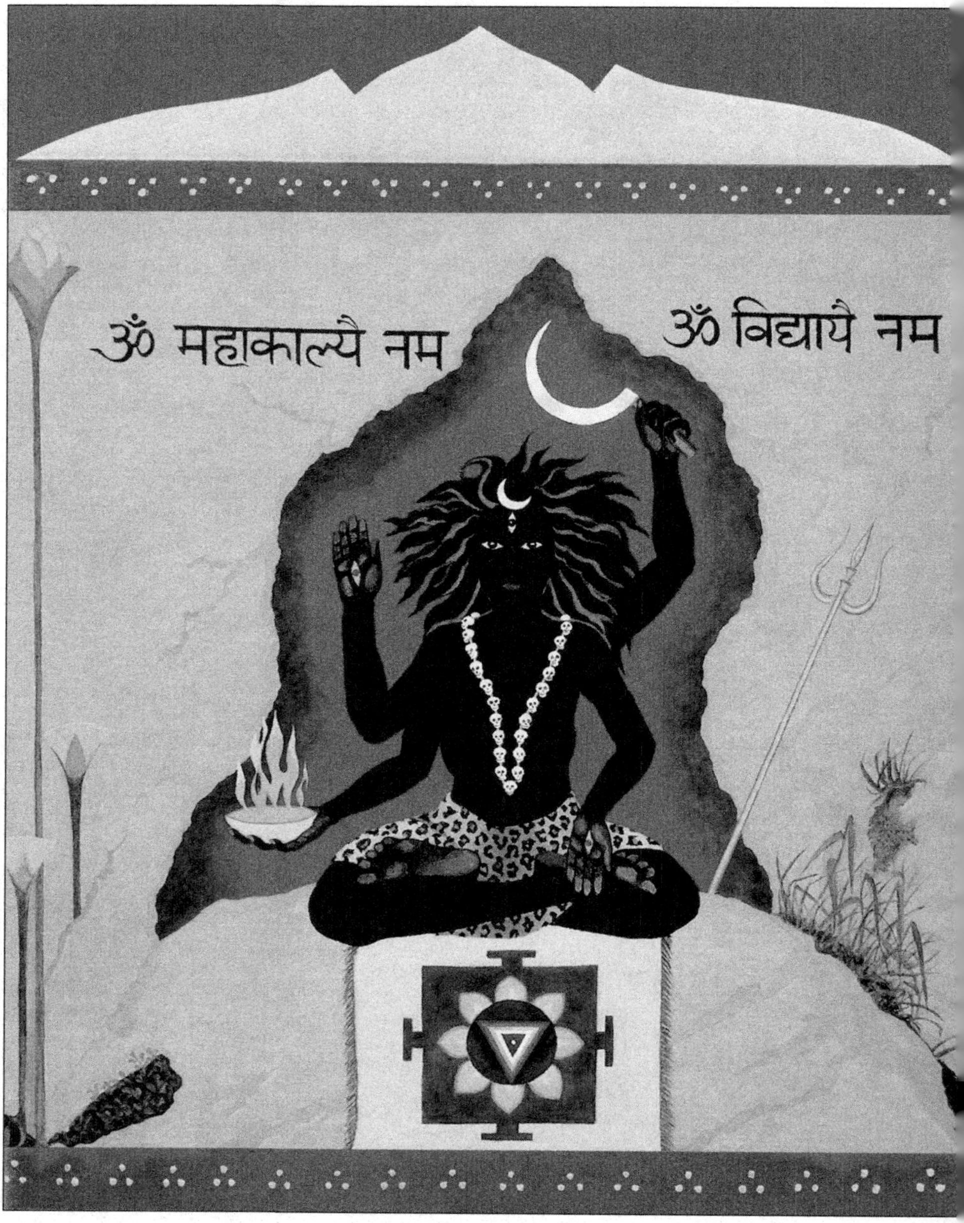

6. Kālī Mahāvidyā, Kālī the Great Wisdom

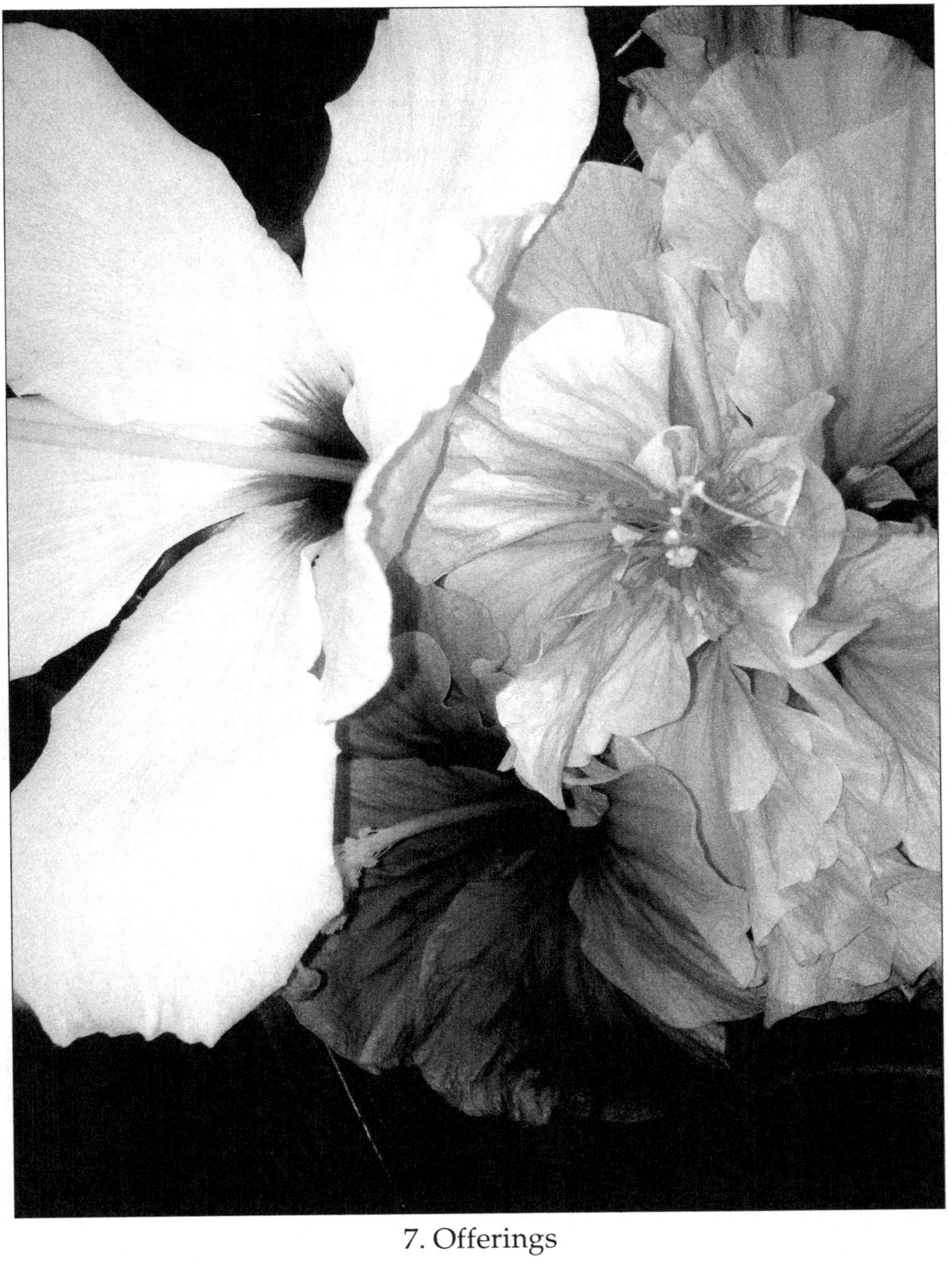

7. Offerings

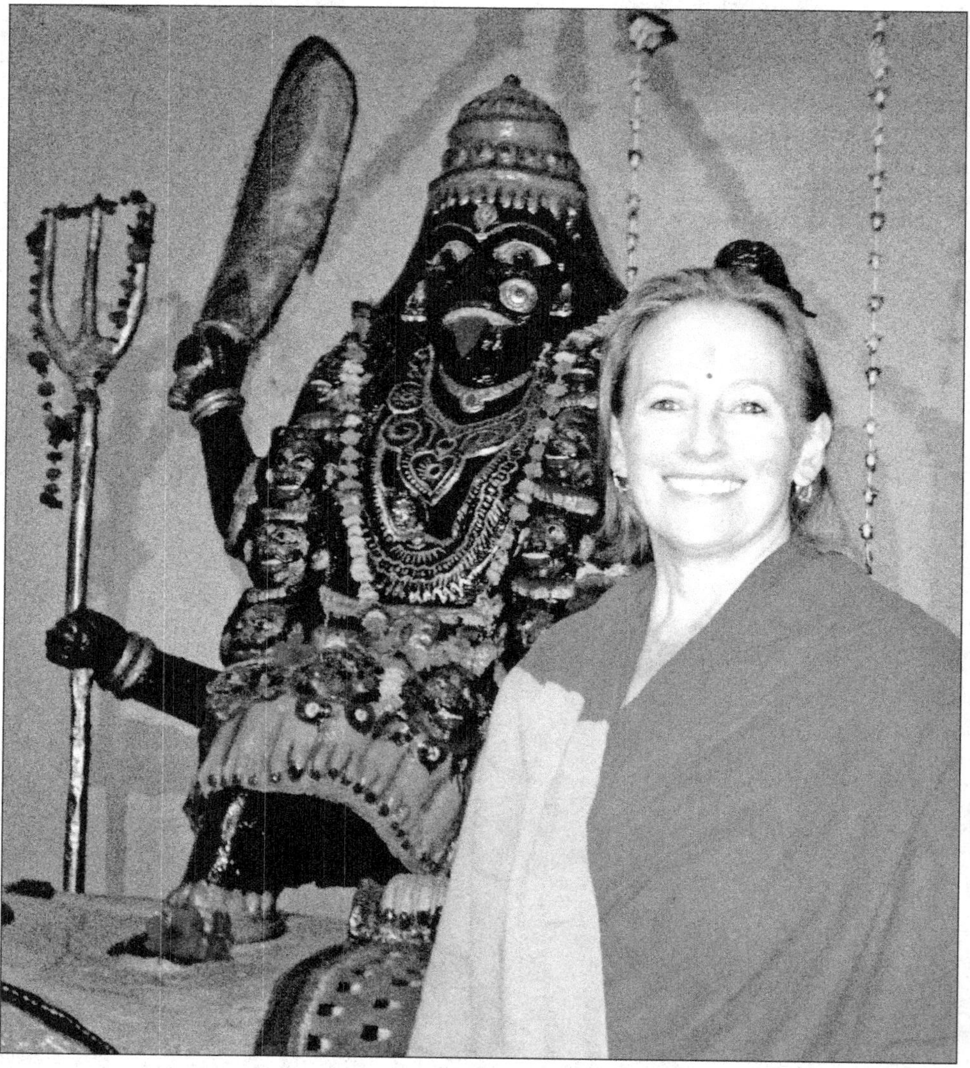

8. Narmadā Kālī has Aditi's head

कालरात्रिः कामरूपा कामपाशविमोचिनी ।
कादम्बिनी कलाधारा कलिकल्मषनाशिनी ॥

kālarātriḥ kāmarūpā kāmapāśavimocinī |
kādambinī kalādhārā kalikalmaṣanāśinī | |

22) Kālarātriḥ (She Who Is the Night of Darkness),
23) Kāmarūpā (She Who Is the Form of Desire),
24) Kāmapāśavimocinī (yet also She Who Is the Liberator from the Bonds of Desire),
25) Kādambinī (She Who Is as Dark as a Bank of Rainclouds),
26) Kalādhārā (She Who Is the Bearer of the Crescent Moon and All Female Energy),
27) Kalikalmaṣanāśinī (She Who Is the Destructress of Evil in the Dark Age of Kālī),

कुमारीपूजनप्रीता कुमारीपूजकालया ।
कुमारीभोजनानन्दा कुमारीरूपधारिणी ॥

kumārīpūjanaprītā kumārīpūjakālayā |
kumārībhojanānandā kumārīrūpadhāriṇī | |

28) Kumārīpūjanaprītā (She Who Loves the Worship of the Virgin-Girls),
29) Kumārīpūjakālayā (She Who Is the Refuge of all Virgin Worshippers),
30) Kumārībhojanānandā (She Who Is Completely Joyed by the Feasts and Gifts to the Virgin-Girls),
31) Kumārīrūpadhāriṇī (She Who Is Herself in the Form of a Virgin-Girl),

कदम्बवनसञ्चारा कदम्बवनवासिनी ।
कदम्बपुष्पसन्तोषा कदम्बपुष्पमालिनी ॥

kadambavanasañcārā kadambavanavāsinī |
kadambapuṣpasantoṣā kadambapuṣpamālinī ||

32) Kadambavanasañcārā (She Who Is a Wanderer [Gopī] in the Kadamba Forest),
33) Kadambavanavāsinī (She Who Is a Dweller in the Kadamba Forest),
34) Kadambapuṣpasantoṣā (She Who Takes Delight in the [Brilliant Yellow] Flowers of the Kadamba Forest),
35) Kadambapuṣpamālinī (She Who Wears a Garland of Kadamba Flowers),

किशोरी कलकण्ठा च कलनादनिनादिनी ।
कादम्बरीपानरता तथा कादम्बरीप्रिया ॥

kiśorī kalakaṇṭhā ca kalanādaninādinī |
kādambarīpānaratā tathā kādambarīpriyā ||

36) Kiśorī (She Who Is Ever Youthful),
37) Kalakaṇṭhā (She Who Has a Soft and Deep-Throated Voice [that Resounds with the Transformative Mantra]), and
38) Kalanādaninādinī (She Who Is Sweet as the Cakravāka Bird),
39) Kādambarīpānaratā (She Who Drinks the Wine-Nectar of the Kādamba Fruit), then
40) Kādambarīpriyā (She Who Is Excited and Pleased with the Kādamba Fruit Wine),

कपालपात्रनिरता कङ्कालमाल्यधारिणी ।
कमलासनसन्तुष्टा कमलासनवासिनी ॥

kapālapātraniratā kaṅkālamālyadhāriṇī |
kamalāsanasantuṣṭā kamalāsanavāsinī | |

41) Kapālapātraniratā (She Who Is Drinking from a Skull Cup),
42) Kaṅkālamālyadhāriṇī (She Who Is Wearing a Garland of Bones),
43) Kamalāsanasantuṣṭā (She Who Is a Lover of the Lotus Flower),
44) Kamalāsanavāsinī (She Who Is Delighted to Be Seated Within the Lotus),

कमलालयमध्यस्था कमलामोदमोदिनी ।
कलहंसगतिः क्लैब्यनाशिनी कामरूपिणी ॥

kamalālayamadhyasthā kamalāmodamodinī |
kalahaṃsagatiḥ klaibyanāśinī kāmarūpiṇī | |

45) Kamalālayamadhyasthā (She Who Is Abiding in the Middle of the Lotus),
46) Kamalāmodamodinī (She Who Is Pleased and Intoxicated by the Scent of the Lotus),
47) Kalahaṃsagatiḥ (She Who Is Moving and Swaying with the Gait of a Black Swan),
48) Klaibyanāśinī (She Who Is the Destroyer of Fears and Iniquity),
49) Kāmarūpiṇī (She Who Is the Form of Desire),

कामरूपकृतावासा कामपीठविलासिनी ।
कमनीया कल्पलता कमनीयविभूषणा ॥

kāmarūpakṛtāvāsā kāmapīṭhavilāsinī |
kamanīyā kalpalatā kamanīyavibhūṣaṇā ||

50) Kāmarūpakṛtāvāsā (She Who Is Residing at Kāmarūpa, the Very Form of Desire),
51) Kāmapīṭhavilāsinī (She Who Is Playing at the Kāmākhyā *Pīṭha*, the Center of the Worship of Desire),
52) Kamanīyā (She Who Is Desired),
53) Kalpalatā (She Who Is the Creeper Who Provides Every Desire),
54) Kamanīyavibhūṣaṇā (She Whose Beauty Is the Ornament),

कमनीयगुणाराध्या कोमलाङ्गी कृशोदरी ।
कारणामृतसन्तोषा कारणानन्दसिद्धिदा ॥

kamanīyaguṇārādhyā komalāṅgī kṛśodarī |
kāraṇāmṛtasantoṣā kāraṇānandasiddhidā ||

55) Kamanīyaguṇārādhyā (She Who Is Pleased with the Quality of Tenderness, She Who Is Worshipped with the Quality of Tenderness),
56) Komalāṅgī (She Who Is Tender-Bodied),
57) Kṛśodarī (She Who Is Slender-Waisted),
58) Kāraṇāmṛtasantoṣā (She Who Is the Cause of the Nectar of Consecrated Wine and is also Pleased with It),
59) Kāraṇānandasiddhidā (She Who Gives *Siddhi* to Those Who Rejoice in Consecrated Wine),

कारणानन्दजापेष्टा कारणार्चनहर्षिता ।
कारणार्णवसम्मग्ना कारणव्रतपालिनी ॥

kāraṇānandajāpeṣṭā kāraṇārcanaharṣitā |
kāraṇārṇavasammagnā kāraṇavratapālinī | |

60) Kāraṇānandajāpeṣṭā (She Who Is the Deity of Those Who Do *Japa* when Joyed with Consecrated Wine),
61) Kāraṇārcanaharṣitā (She Who Is Glad to be Worshipped with Consecrated Wine),
62) Kāraṇārṇavasammagnā (She Who Is Immersed in an Ocean of Consecrated Wine),
63) Kāraṇavratapālinī (She Who Protects Those Who Accomplish *Vrata* with Consecrated Wine),

कस्तूरीसौरभामोदा कस्तूरीतिलकोज्ज्वला ।
कस्तूरीपूजनरता कस्तूरीपूजकप्रिया ॥

kastūrīsaurabhāmodā kastūrītilakojjvalā |
kastūrīpūjanaratā kastūrīpūjakapriyā | |

64) Kastūrīsaurabhāmodā (She Who Is Gladdened by the Scent of Musk),
65) Kastūrītilakojjvalā (She Who Is the Luminous One with a *Tīlaka* of Musk),
66) Kastūrīpūjanaratā (She Who Rejoices in the Worship with Musk),
67) Kastūrīpūjakapriyā (She Who Loves Those Who Worship Her with Musk),

कस्तूरीदाहजननी कस्तूरीमृगतोषिणी ।
कस्तूरीभोजनप्रीता कर्पूरामोदमोदिता ।
कर्पूरमालाभरणा कर्पूरचन्दनोक्षिता ॥

kastūrīdāhajananī kastūrīmṛgatoṣiṇī |
kastūrībhojanaprītā karpūrāmodamoditā |
karpūramālābharaṇā karpūracandanokṣitā | |

68) Kastūrīdāhajananī (She Who Is Mother of Those Who Burn Musk as Incense),
69) Kastūrīmṛgatoṣiṇī (She Who Is Fond of the Musk Deer),
70) Kastūrībhojanaprītā (She Who Is Pleased to Eat the Musk of the Musk Deer),
71) Karpūrāmodamoditā (She Who Is Gladdened by the Scent of Camphor),
72) Karpūramālābharaṇā (She Who Is Adorned with Garlands of Camphor),
73) Karpūracandanokṣitā (She Whose Body Is Smeared with Camphor and Sandalpaste),

कर्पूरकारणाह्लादा कर्पूरामृतपायिनी ।
कर्पूरसागरस्नाता कर्पूरसागरालया ॥

karpūrakāraṇāhlādā karpūrāmṛtapāyinī |
karpūrasāgarasnātā karpūrasāgarālayā | |

74) Karpūrakāraṇāhlādā (She Who Is Pleased with Consecrated Wine with Camphor),
75) Karpūrāmṛtapāyinī (She Who Drinks the Nectar with Camphor),
76) Karpūrasāgarasnātā (She Who Is Bathed in the Ocean of Camphor),
77) Karpūrasāgarālayā (She Who Is at Home in the Ocean of Camphor),

कूर्चबीजजपप्रीता कूर्चजापपरायणा ।
कुलीना कौलिकाराध्या कौलिकप्रियकारिणी ॥

kūrcabījajapaprītā kūrcajāpaparāyaṇā ।
kulīnā kaulikārādhyā kaulikapriyakāriṇī ।।

78) Kūrcabījajapaprītā (She Who Is Pleased When Worshipped with the Recitation of the Bīja *Hūṁ*),
79) Kūrcajāpaparāyaṇā (She Who Threatens and Conquers Demons by Muttering *Hūṁ*),
80) Kulīnā (She Who Is the Embodiment of the Kulācāra, the Kula Teachings),
81) Kaulikārādhyā (She Who Is Adored by Kaulika, the Practitioners of the Kulācāra),
82) Kaulikapriyakāriṇī (She Who Is the Benefactress of the Kaulika, the Cause of the Love [of the Kaulika for the Kulācāra]),

कुलाचारा कौतुकिनी कुलमार्गप्रदर्शिनी ।
काशीश्वरी कष्टहर्त्री काशीशवरदायिनी ॥

kulācārā kautukinī kulamārgapradarśinī ।
kāśīśvarī kaṣṭahartrī kāśīśavaradāyinī ।।

83) Kulācārā (She Who Is Observant of the Kulācāra),
84) Kautukinī (She Who Is the Joyous One),
85) Kulamārgapradarśinī (She Who Is the Revealer of the Kula Path to Seekers),
86) Kāśīśvarī (She Who Is the Supreme Goddess of Kāśī-Varanasi),
87) Kaṣṭahartrī (She Who Removes Difficulties, Suffering),
88) Kāśīśavaradāyinī (She Who Is the Giver of Blessings to Śiva, Lord of Kāśī-Varanasi),

काशीश्वरकृतामोदा काशीश्वरमनोरमा ॥

kāśīśvarakṛtāmodā kāśīśvaramanoramā | |

89) Kāśīśvarakṛtāmodā (She Who Is the Giver of Pleasure to the Lord of Kāśī),
90) Kāśīśvaramanoramā (She Who Is the Beloved of the Lord of Kāśī, She Who Overwhelms His Mind with Beauty),

कलमञ्जीरचरणा क्वणत्काञ्चीविभूषणा ।
काञ्चनाद्रिकृतागारा काञ्चनाचलकौमुदी ॥

kalamañjīracaraṇā kvaṇatkāñcīvibhūṣaṇā |
kāñcanādrikṛtāgārā kāñcanācalakaumudī | |

91) Kalamañjīracaraṇā (She Whose Toe Bells Make Sweet Melodies as She Moves),
92) Kvaṇatkāñcīvibhūṣaṇā (She Whose Girdle Bells Sweetly Tinkle),
93) Kāñcanādrikṛtāgārā (She Who Is Residing in the Golden Mountain, Mount Meru),
94) Kāñcanācalakaumudī (She Who Is the Shining Moonbeam on the Mountain of Gold, She Who Displays Radiant Wealth on Her Top Cloth),

कामबीजजपानन्दा कामबीजस्वरूपिणी ।
कुमतिघ्नी कुलीनार्तिनाशिनी कुलकामिनी ॥

kāmabījajapānandā kāmabījasvarūpiṇī |
kumatighnī kulīnārtināśinī kulakāminī ||

95) Kāmabījajapānandā (She Who Is in Complete Bliss to Hear the Recitation of the Bīja Mantra *Klīṃ*),
96) Kāmabījasvarūpiṇī (She Who Is the Embodiment of the Bīja Mantra *Klīṃ*, She Who Is the Form of the Kāma Bīja),
97) Kumatighnī (She Who Is the Destroyer of all Evil Inclinations),
98) Kulīnārtināśinī (She Who Is the Destroyer of the Afflictions of the Kaulika),
99) Kulakāminī (She Who Is the Entire Family of Desires, She Who Is the Lady of the Kula, the Kaulas),

क्रीं ह्रीं श्रीं मन्त्रवर्णेन कालकण्टकघातिनी ।
इत्याद्याकालिकादेव्याः शतनाम प्रकीर्तितम् ॥

krīṃ hrīṃ śrīṃ mantravarṇena kālakaṇṭakaghātinī |
ityādyākālikādevyāḥ śatanāma prakīrtitam ||

100) I make obeisance to Kālakaṇṭakaghātinī, She Who Is by the Bīja, *Krīṃ, Hrīṃ, Śrīṃ*, the Destroyer of the Fear of Death.
These are known as the Hundred Names of Devī Ādyā Kālikā,

ककारकूटघटितं कालीरूपस्वरूपकम् ॥

kakārakūṭaghaṭitaṃ kālīrūpasvarūpakam ||

beginning with the letter KA. They are all identical with the form of Kālī.

III.
CONTEMPLATIONS OF ĀDYĀ KĀLĪ'S HUNDRED NAMES

Contemplations of Ādyā Kālī's Hundred Names

As you undertake a nightly practice of the *Song of the Hundred Names of Ādyā Kālī* and begin your journey with the Contemplations of Her Hundred Names, you will notice a decided focus on Ādyā Kālī's names from the point of view of the female practitioner, the yoginī. If you are in a male body, a transgendered body, or a non-gendered body, this should not deter you. This practice can be undertaken by anyone; all forms are her forms. All are welcome here. In this lineage, the physical form of our body is not a limitation. We practice into the depths of whatever form we have, and arise from within that, knowing that we are Kālī, we are her. The *Song of the Hundred Names of Ādyā Kālī* is a powerful teaching on how any form that incarnates is her.

You who have incarnated in a female body (whether you have a physical womb-yoni or not) will find yourselves drawn dynamically into your own feminine embodiment through these contemplations. Know yourself *as her* in all these potentially new and unexpected ways.

Those in male bodies, multi-gendered, transgendered bodies, and/or non-gendered bodies, will likely experience the depths of your own internal feminine energies (whether you have a physical womb-yoni or not), and come into greater healing and wholeness, more readily able to express this part of yourself.

You will hopefully find an entryway into loving devotion and reverence for the feminine in all her forms. In turn, your masculine energies will be attended to in many subtle ways. Your own wholeness will emerge as a result.

As you undertake a nightly practice of reciting the *Song of the Hundred Names of Ādyā Kālī*, it is important not to jump around or jump ahead. Please read just one contemplation each night. For more details on this rationale, please refer back to Chapter 9 of the Introduction.

1) *Hrīṃ* Kālī

The first three names hold Tantric paradoxical mysteries, and I'll point these out as we go through each contemplation; they build on each other here. For today, hold Kālī as Ādyā Kālī as her seed syllable *hrīṃ*. It is relevant that, in the *Song of the Hundred Names of Ādyā Kālī*, we find that Kālī, the first name, is *hrīṃ*—the bīja mantra associated with birth and becoming. Traditionally, it is far more common for Kālī to be associated with either *krīṃ* or perhaps *klīṃ*. Here, Kālī is she who births the cosmos, Ādyā Kālī, the primordial cosmic Kālī. The first name is the birthing. We have begun.

As you practice today, attune to the vibration of birth in your body and in your practice. Find some way to resonate with the sounds and the experience. Bring gentle regard to the newness and the tender shoots of potential that are sprouting. This wellspring of birthing aliveness is our Ādyā Kālī Mā. This Ādyā Kālī brings the unconscious into consciousness, the unmanifest into the manifest.

2) *Śrīṃ* Karālī (She Who Is Formidable, Dreadful)

The three bīja mantras of these first three contemplations of Ādyā Kālī's hundred names are linked in the cycle of birthing, sustaining, and transforming. As noted above, normally Kālī is associated with the bīja *krīṃ* and transformation. Here though, the Tantric mysteries begin at the beginning. Yesterday, it was Ādyā Kālī giving birth to the universe via the bīja mantra *hrīṃ* as the first name in our recitation. Tonight, night two, it is another fierce goddess, Karālī, who offers preservation and sustaining energies. As I do, you can consider: How might a terrifying Devī bring sustaining and preserving energies? How might such formidable energies serve us ongoingly?

As for what Karālī looks like and where her temples are, in this form there is almost no information about her. Karālī is a mystery to be revealed through our presencing with her. What is your experience of her?

3) *Krīṃ* Kalyāṇī (She Who Is the Bestower of Wellbeing)

The mysteries continue to unfold here with this name . . . the bīja mantra *krīṃ* is the manifestation of transformation and death; it is about letting things die and move down into the fertile darkness. There is a fullness in *krīṃ* though, the way a decaying compost heap has fullness in it. The cast offs, discards, and end bits are transforming into something that will eventually emerge as a rich fertile matrix.

This *krīṃ* in the third name salutes and is linked to Kalyāṇī, the bestower of peace and happiness. Death and transformation linked to peace and happiness: a profound wisdom teaching.

In these first three names we can see the inseparability of all her aspects. There is no clear and easy correspondence of the names, their qualities, and the form in which they emerge. What is universally true though is that Kālī can hold all of this mystery and paradox until it unfolds in each of us as wisdom.

Kalyāṇī also has a relationship to the subtle body, and an inner process that requires us to bring love and awareness into our bodies more fully. In turn, we cultivate our willingness to turn towards bodily sensation and experience. The causal body is the energetic body, or matrix (note that "body" is far too strong and concrete a word for what is actually being referred to here), that *causes* the subtle body to come into manifestation. Our subtle body is made up of an entire web of winds and channels and śakti that infuse our physical form and are intertwined with it. All of these delicate vital energetics arise as a result of the matrix of the causal body, which is even more subtle and ephemeral, and is the source and resting place of some of the deepest wisdom inherent in embodiment. This wisdom is just waiting to overwhelm us with the bliss of awakening in the body, in this lifetime. Bliss and consciousness, love and awareness, are our true nature.

Kālī, as the qualities of peace and happiness (dare we say *bliss*?), allows the subtle body to dissolve into the causal body at the time of death. Thus we return to her, we dissolve into her irrevocably, once again. The spiritual practices that reveal this inherent bliss and awareness in the body are a vital part of the Kālīkula. What are those practices? For now, please rest with that question, knowing that the answers will unfold.

May peace and happiness arise as wisdom in your body. May Kalyāṇī show us the way. Don't forget to take notes in your journal about your experience with Kalyāṇī.

4) Kalāvatī (She Who Is the Possessor of the [64] Arts)

Kalāvatī takes us into the fourth night of the recitation of the *Song of the Hundred Names of Ādyā Kālī*. With this name, we come to the end of the first Sanskrit line in the *stotra*.* The door that is revealed to us through the recitation of the bīja mantras of the first three names is flung wide open into the fourth name. Full and complete with the entire cycle of birth/generation, preservation/sustaining, and death/transformation, we come full stop to Kalāvatī who possesses the Sixty-four Arts.

The Sixty-four Arts refer to the sixty-four "intimate acts of worship" or the sixty-four forms of desire, or the sixty-four yoginīs. Each of the sixty-four yoginīs in the circle holds full and complete embodiment and wisdom of one of the arts—a full chakra in complete display; the bīja in full cycling with the energy of sacred desire to enliven it all.

Kalāvatī is the bindu, the coalescing centerpoint, who, through her possession of them, gathers all the yoginīs and all the intimate arts/acts into herself. She is the matrix of energy that moves all the forms of desire into our daily spiritual practice. When we consider Kalāvatī and the Sixty-four Arts in the same heartbeat, what is revealed is the Tantric teaching of the multiplicity as the one, and the one as the multiplicity. The microcosm as the macrocosm, macrocosm as microcosm. These energies move back and forth, in and out, like the tides or the moon phases. Kalāvatī disperses into the sixty-four in full radiant display. The sixty-four are then gathered up and merge into Kalāvatī as one. This is the ebb and flow of līlā. This is the ebb and flow of the cosmos. This is the ebb and flow of moon blood and desire. Here, with Kalāvatī, this līlā is inherent.

I surrender to that form of Kālī that is all the Sixty-four Acts of intimate worship. I prostrate to that Kalāvatī who applies a tantalizing flirt to bring us into relationship with and commitment to our spiritual practices. I bow before the Sixty-four Arts that allow the fullest expression of awakening in this body in this lifetime. As one of my teachers offered, the Tantric path is far more an art than a science.

At this point I will restrain myself from offering specifics, or lists, of the Sixty-four Arts. There is no need to bring more complexity to this spiritual practice than is necessary now. In addition, it's far more interesting for you to contemplate and compose your own lists. Just as the lists of the names of the sixty-four yoginīs varies from text to text, inscription to inscription, temple to temple, so too do the other lists flux and flow. They arise in different locations, times, and contexts, to meet the needs of her worshippers. Kālī arises in the form that we need her, right now. I need Kalāvatī in the form that she arises for me, today.

Journal a little about the sixty-four forms of *your* sacred desire, as you wish. Wearing Kalāvatī's form today, move into the world *as* desire, as the yoginī who has perfected desire as a blessing for all beings. What happens?

May we know Kalāvatī's Sixty-four Arts and acts of worship through our own experience. May her desire bless our desire.

5) Kamalā (She Who Is the Lotus)

There is so much richness and layering in each of her names that my entire inner landscape is already changed, alight, humming. Everything is different. Already. I felt this change initially a few weeks ago when I undertook a new practice to prepare for this commitment to the recitation of her names. I felt it coming together yesterday in my body in a new way with Kalāvatī and her Sixty-four Arts. Kalāvatī's desire moves as openness, and the world is responding. I feel my habitual bodily constriction, as well as the glory of openness and love flowing.

The first three names with the bīja mantras describe the unceasing cyclic nature of the yoniverse. The forms of desire in the fourth name are the power source for this unceasing nature. We then have the activity of all existence, as well as the energies that animate the activity.

The fifth name, Kamalā, then arises. The question is not "Who is Kamalā, the Lotus One?" but "What and where is this lotus in relation to the yoniverse that is being mapped in the *Song of the Hundred Names of Ādyā Kālī?*" "Where is this lotus that enjoys and is enjoyed?" It is the womb that is the location, or seat, of the deity in a woman's body maṇḍala. The generative organs in the pelvis are the center of the body in this worldview, not the heart as is common in many spiritual traditions. The heart is important, indeed, it's just not the seat of power. In this tradition we spend time cultivating desire, and moving the center of gravity from our heart down into our pelvis, into the yoni (which is comprised of the outer genitalia as well as the vaginal canal, the cervix, the uterus, and the fallopian tubes). We live from the yoni. In the center of the yoni is the cervix— the soft, regal, undulating seat and home of Kālī, at least during this sādhana. Kālī as Kamalā indicates that Kālī is taking her seat in my womb. Kālī pervades from there.

As she who enjoys and is enjoyed, Kamalā-Kālī gestures towards the mystery of the cultivation of desire. In the union practices in this lineage, the cervix is the focus of our attention as female practitioners. This is not to say that we ignore the other parts of the yoni. We worship the entire yoni! Yet, if we had to choose a central point, a bindu, it would be the cervix. Perhaps you can begin to enjoy the sensations that arise from the cervix for yourself? Maybe put your hands on your pelvis, your generative organs, and feel the power pulsing here, the raw power of existence.

When I discuss desire, I'm not talking about regular sexual desire (although that is included), but instead about the kind of desire that activates feminine and masculine polarities in ourselves and in the outer world, and then allows us to skillfully merge those polarities into union. Desire is the powerhouse of energy that fuels this potent merging. Desire offers the potential for union, two as one. This union can happen just within myself, or it can happen between myself and another being.

Perhaps you can spend time today feeling the energies of your generative organs. Can you explore the energy of the presence of the lotus of your cervix that is Kamalā, Kālī's seat? Journal a little about the nature of your own desire: its ways, textures, nuances, its ebb and flow. If you knew that your cervix was the center of your being, how would that change how you relate to yourself and the world?

6) Kalidarpaghnī (She Who Destroys Pride during the Kālī Yuga)

Kalidarpaghnī stands watch over the tendency towards too much pride during the *Kālī Yuga;* she keeps it in check during this age in which it is likely to run rampant. Why destroy pride? We all know there are unhealthy types of pride, and yet with self-awareness we might wonder "isn't a little pride a good thing, a kind of self-love and indication of self-worth?" Indeed, it might be, and yet there is something more subtle being gestured towards, in true Tantric fashion. Kalidarpaghnī is the form of Kālī who also gestures towards what is obscured by pride. In pride there is little room for the grace of devotional surrender and trust to emerge. Kalidarpaghnī thus takes away what keeps us from union with her.

Surrender is a tricky topic, and self-inquiry will benefit here. With Kālī's support, I suggest that you investigate your attitudes towards devotional surrender. What are you willing to surrender to? What are you willing to bow to? What are your assumptions about surrender? What is your own experience or lack or experience in the domain of surrender? Might you risk asking Kalidarpaghnī-Kālī to destroy your pride? What would then have the room to emerge?

I've been referring directly and indirectly to being one with Mā, being in union. Identification with Mā, Devī, Kālī, the deity, allows us the opportunity to cultivate authentic self-esteem and self-worth. Not puffed up and assertive, not boastful, not prideful. Instead, a union that emerges from an inner knowing. This is not in contrast or opposition to devotional surrender as it might seem upon first investigation: it goes hand in hand with it.

Our devotional surrender allows an opening to a path of union with Kālī, an authentic understanding of divine service (*seva**) that is not based on any standards of assessment you or others may hold (*Look at how well I did that! Oh I had the 2AM* *shift. I did _____. They couldn't have done it without me, it wouldn't happen without me. Good job! Well done!* and on and on). Perhaps you might experiment with dropping all notions that you know what devotional surrender or service/offering are. Do some anonymous seva and find out. Don't get prideful about your accomplishment (inwardly or outwardly). Instead, rest in knowing that you are melting away all in you that separates you from her. Let hard work in service to others melt you. Kalidarpaghnī is your ally in this.

7) Kapardīśakṛpānvitā (She Who Gives Grace to the One of Matted Hair)

Seven names complete our first week together. Seven names complete the first stanza of this most precious liturgy. Kapardīśakṛpānvitā is the final name in the first stanza and describes Kālī's influence on her consort Śiva; she gives him grace.

So inseparable are Kālī in Śiva that, even in such a goddess-oriented liturgy as the *Song of the Hundred Names of Ādyā Kālī*, we find that Śiva and his matted hair shows up as the completion name. In terms of the overall logic of this stanza, the first three names establish the name of the mystery of how manifestation occurs, wrapped in the mysteries of Kālī's forms as birth/preservation/transformation. We then move to desire—the energy that animates all existence. After that, Kālī-Kamalā points to *where* in our bodies this work of the cosmos takes place. Then, it is Kalidarpaghnī's melting away of inaccurate pride that allows devotional surrender. This attitude, along with the movement of desire is what allows the grace of Kālī's communion with Śiva to emerge: union. Almost all the mysteries of the path are unveiled in this first stanza. The remaining stanzas and ninety-three names are the reiteration of the themes we find here, right at the beginning.

Śiva of the matted hair is usually understood as the fierce form of Śiva. This is fierce union indeed. Śiva has grace because of

Kālī as Kapardīśakṛpānvitā. Her grace infuses him, is a blessing force in his existence, in much the same way that women are understood as blessing forces to men in this lineage.

As you wish, take a few minutes to journal about the specific nature of your own feminine grace. Can you sense how your body is a blessing force, is the movement of grace in the world? Can you sense how you might offer grace to others in your world? In addition, explore the logic of this first stanza by writing a sentence or two about your movement through the names, and how the themes emerge for you. This kind of linking of your inner experiences to the liturgy will support you in making the *Song of the Hundred Names of Ādyā Kālī* your own.

8) Kālikā (She Who Is the Devourer of Time)

We begin the second stanza with the eighth name and our attention turns away from the intimacy of Kapardīśakṛpānvitā-Kālī in grace and union with fierce Śiva. Our focus now is the movement towards a form of Kālī that is larger than even space and time: Kālikā. Just as time devours our lives, moment by moment, so too does Kālikā in turn devour even that devouring time. Everything comes forth from her womb and she devours it as well, bringing it all back into herself. As Kālikā, she is the cyclic nature of it all, once again.

This name shows us how intimacy with her can be small and personal, where we sense all the minutiae, or large and all encompassing. It can be generative lovemaking in one breath and the death of time in the next. There is only an inhale, an exhale, and the retention of the space after the two breaths, between these two aspects of Kālīkā-Kālī. This macrocosmic/microcosmic worldview is a potent training.

On another level, this Kālikā who devours that devouring time is also pointing to a state of realization that is beyond time, that transcends time. Even when time is gone, she will be there as the matrix of all of this. Resting in her, with her, allows us to rest in what continues even when life as we know it ends.

How about wearing all black today in honor of Kālikā? Then, every time you see the color black around you, note it as her presence.

I rejoice in this Kālikā as the truth there is, beyond all conception.

9) Kālamātā (She Who Is Mother of Time)

Kālamātā holds this minute-vastness within herself as the mother of time and the destroyer of time. She is the matrix that exists before all markers of existence, before any manifestation, and then she births it all through her formless body. This body is also what destroys time, taking it all back into herself. Like many other Śākta goddesses, she offers both existence and non-existence. She gives form to the unformed, and from form she draws us back into her womb where we rest in nonduality.

Her cosmic womb birthing time, birthing mortality, is not separate from our wombs. Like Kālamātā, our wombs also offer birth and move death. Our wombs bring forth manifest existence, just as hers does.

With this dual awareness of before-time and the death of time, can you bring your inner knowing to how Kālamātā is drawing *you* further into her womb? How she draws you into your own womb and generative organs? Can you sense that galaxies are coming into existence in the mouth of your cervix? Do you experience the giving of death as your moon blood passes out? What is alive because of your yoni-womb? What has died, is dying, as a result of the cosmic matrix of your yoni-womb? If there is anything to rejoice in with all of this, make offerings to Kālamātā. If there is anything to grieve, make offerings to Kālamātā.

10) Kālānalasamadyutiḥ (She Who Is as Radiant as the Fires That Consume the Universe)

First dark and now bright: Kālī shifts and changes as quickly as our subtle moods and flows (which, of course, she is not separate from). Kālānalasamadyutiḥ shows us that when death comes, as it always does, fire consumes it all.

In this radiant brightness, we can ask ourselves what the nature of feminine radiance is, and what is its source. Reference your own body as you address these questions.

In my own experience, this incredible radiance of Kālānalasamadyutiḥ-Kālī comes from openness, from softness; a kind of emotional and bodily availability. This availability allows śakti to move freely, and out into the world, so that radiance also can be felt and experienced by others.

Another form of this blazing radiance is experienced when we are so in love with goddess that we are truly and literally on fire. Ablaze with the fires of her. What awful delight! This is the radiant blaze that burns away everything that is not her, leaving only her behind. This process is not always pretty, and is surely messy. Yet for those of us burning in this way, there is no dousing this fire, nor walking away from it. There is no place we'd rather be except standing here in her radiance until the blaze is so bright that it consumes the universe. We return to her. This is Kālānalasamadyutiḥ.

Can you sense how feminine radiance, and being, and her radiance are related? When was the last time you knew yourself as radiant? How did you arrive there? When was the last time you stood in the devotional fires burning with your love for her? Have you ever loved so hot and wild that you were almost consumed by it? What emerged on the other side?

Let this be a day for referencing your body wisdom. Can you explore and reference gratitude for the body temple that you have, that you are? This is the temple. This is the pilgrimage.

11) Kapardinī (She Who Has Matted Hair)

Such praise to she who wears matted hair, the dreadlocks. This matted hair shows that she is close to, inseparable from, Śiva with the matted locks. Among spiritual practitioners, dreadlocks are a sign of living at the edges of social life, outside normal conventions. They are a sign of living in devotion to the divine, outside of household life.

Dreadlocks are seen as a natural arising when the kuṇḍalinī begins to move in our bodies. The energy of Śakti intensifies and swirls as desire in the yoni-womb. The matted hair is her snake body, the movement of grace through us bringing bliss, freedom, awareness, and awakening.

Can you sense how Kapardinī might be the secret practitioner? The woman wearing dreadlocks (perhaps just one or two secret ones), who is inseparable from Śiva, and the woman with kuṇḍalinī energies moving through her?

Yesterday with Kālānalasamadyutih we referenced radiant energy. Today, we can consider for ourselves where in the body this radiance of union with Śiva might arise? Where in the body does kuṇḍalinī arise? Can you feel these energies? There is indeed more than one mood or texture of energy here. I invite you to journal about these energies, and where and how they live in *your* body. Perhaps you might draw and color a picture of this energy in motion, instead of writing about it. Let yourself dive into your subtle world, holding Kapardinī-Kālī in your mind's eye, and notice what arises.

12) Karālāsyā (She Who Has Fangs and a Formidable Expression)

We have just begun to taste the essence of Kapardinī and now we are moving on. *It's too fast,* I cry! But Karālāsyā's fierce countenance, her fierce mood, tells me there is no possibility of slowing down. Truly we are going at lightning speed. The fierce and formidable stance of Karālāsyā lets us know we are undertaking serious business with the investigation of Ādyā Kālī's forms. Truth and awakening are not always tidy, pretty, or sweet. Coming to terms with Karālāsyā-Kālī's fierce side is part of the embrace of everything that allows union to emerge and stabilize. If we turn towards the soft and gentle, and yet push away the hard and fierce, we are pushing away the entirety of ways she manifests and only allowing a partial view. Awakening requires the whole view. Karālāsyā holds us to that.

What emerges for us when we turn towards her fierce face, her fierce posture? What do you learn about your preferences from this movement towards her? Can you also sense your own strength and courage emerge in the face of her formidableness? This is the courage and strength that we need on this path. Her formidableness is training for our own endurance on the Tantric path. Meet her and you will be able to meet everything that will come forth as a result of practice, everything in life actually. Can you meet Karālāsyā eye to eye here? If you find yourself reticent about this, turn towards yourself with love, and inquire about what is happening. Investigate that reticence, without judgment, knowing you are being held by Karālāsyā-Kālī with great love in the process.

13) Karuṇāmṛtasāgarā (yet also She Who Is the Oceanic Nectar of Compassion)

We come to the last name in the second stanza with Karuṇāmṛtasāgarā. Karālāsyā's fierce countenance (including a gaping mouth, according to some sources) confronts us with some of the darker aspects of the path. Yet she now merges with Karuṇāmṛtasāgarā, she who is the ocean of the nectar of compassion. Do you know that Kālī's fierceness is simultaneously compassionate? Her compassion is so true that it produces nectar, *amṛta,** and in endless oceanic quantities. This is her ever constant love and compassion for our human existence. The primordial expression of she is a love so vast and fierce and full of compassion that it extends beyond all our notions and experiences of space, time, possibility. This is Ādyā Kālī before form and manifestation: endless, sweet, oceanic nectar. When she manifests, this nectar pours forth into all existence, bathing us in healing, nourishing, and enlivening essences.

On a more personal level, can you imagine *yourself* as the source of a nectar of compassion, and with oceanic amounts of it? What if this nectar, amṛta, emerged from your nether mouth? That is, what if your generative organs were the source of this nectar? Could you identify with Kālī's wisdom so that your own body fluids were not separate from hers, but instead a result of your union with her? Can you imagine your sexual fluids and moon blood as sacred? And if so, what is the compassion inherent therein? Can you bring gentle regard to your experience of your sexual fluids and moon blood as Karuṇāmṛtasāgarā-Kālī's?

Big questions, I know. What is your body sensation in response?

14) Kṛpāmayī (She Who Is Full of Grace)

We come to the end of the second stanza today, and the end of the second week of reciting her names. Is there a rhythm developing and moving through you with recitation of the names? Do you sense how each name is connected to the one before and the one after, and how each stanza has its own cohesion. Can you feel her mercy, Kṛpāmayī's mercy and grace, moving in you through the recitation of the names?

For me, there is a thread of śakti in the recitation of her names, an opening to the river of grace that flows from immersion in her sacred waters. I know she is near and I feel Kṛpāmayī-Kālī's grace manifesting. Remarkably, I have both an inner embodied taste of Mā's grace as well as the experience of it manifesting externally.

In this process, I have been dropping into and reflecting on the intimate and ongoing relationship of the microcosmic and the macrocosmic-aspects of the yoniverse. Can you feel that too?

In what ways might Kṛpāmayī-Kālī's mercy and grace be coming to birth in your body and in your external world? For what do you need more mercy and grace in your life? Gently place your inner awareness on how gratitude supports the movement of grace and mercy. The movement of grace is intimately connected to stabilizing in love and awareness, bliss and consciousness. Do you experience this, in any way, in your body? Can you feel this in others? Can you move your love and awareness from the intimate details of your subtle body and inner world out into the cosmos? If not, perhaps pray for more grace. If so, keep praying!

15) Kṛpādhārā (She Who Is the Vessel of Mercy, the Supporter of Grace)

Go carefully dear ones, go carefully. Take a little rest today and tomorrow, in Kālī Mā's grace. It's time for some extra self-care, and nourishment. Go *slooooowly* right now. We are at an edge, a precipice, and it never hurts to pause before we jump again. And we *will* be jumping again. Hopefully to fly.

Yesterday, today, and tomorrow, we contemplate and experience the grace of resting in her mercy. Things will unfold and unwind as we rest down, and that's perfect. Let them, and schedule extra time to appreciate this winding down. Sometimes we unconsciously slip into illness or injury to make the space we need to truly rest at the level that her practices require. There is no blame here; I say this for myself too. Proceed with extra care. Ask for help. Give yourself time to integrate. A few extra shrine offerings would be beneficial today. I will be doing just that on behalf of all of us.

Kṛpādhārā is the supporter of grace, the womb-vessel of mercy. Let her offer you some of that right now. Rest. Dream sweetly. Eat with love. Offer love. Receive love. That's enough, you know.

Just as the yoni-womb brings forth compassion, it is also the home of grace and mercy. If you can, find this home of compassion in yourself, in your body. Otherwise, just rest into knowing it is true, and that Mā has you in this.

16) Kṛpāpārā (She Whose Mercy Is Without Limit, She Who Is Beyond Grace)

Different flavors of Ādyā Kālī are expressed in this current run of her names. We went from a fierce face—with Karālāsyā—to the ocean of the nectar of compassion. We basked in grace and mercy coming into manifestation for our benefit with our sinking into Kṛpāmayī. Then, yesterday, we discovered the bodily location of this manifestation: the vessel and supporter of this grace and mercy is Kṛpādhārā's womb, her yoni crucible, inseparable from ours. Today we discover that not only is this grace and mercy manifesting on the micro-level, in our bodies as her body, but that this mercy is unlimited. In this form, Kṛpāpārā-Kālī is so vast that she exceeds all manifest existence. The last three names (including today's) mirror the basic yonic triangulation of creating/sustaining/transforming. This womb of grace is so primordial (these are the names of the primordial Kālī, after all), so beyond our notions of existence, that she is also transformation/destruction. Kālī's nature is unceasing. Are you observing the movement of energy as the names link to each other and flow through each other? Are you sensing that no boundaries exist where one name stops and the next begins?

Continue to let yourself soak up the mercy and grace of her expression, which is infinite. This is the nourishment we need right now. Rest into it and drink it in. Explore it. Do you have any resistance to taking in this much nourishment? Do you think you might not deserve it, that it's not all for you? Actually, it's all for you.

May your devotion burn away all obstacles, transform all adversity. May you be happy. May Kṛpāpārā's mercy and grace enliven you always.

17) Kṛpāgamā (She Who Is Attainable Only by Her Mercy, She Who Moves in Grace)

We are in the last day of this run of names that relate to Kālī's grace and mercy as we come to the end of the first line of this stanza. Take a breath here, the way you do at the end of a sentence—a brief pause, so you can continue to drink in her mercy and grace as nourishment. Can you identify some way her mercy and grace are present and working in your life right now? In addition, notice the wisdom of this grace and mercy, and how it allows for union with her. Kṛpāgamā-Kālī's mercy is a pathway to her. All movement comes from Kṛpāgamā and goes back to her. Know her as your every breath, as the animator of every movement. Never ending. Can you feel this for yourself and cultivate trust in it?

Keep resting as you can today and taking care of the rising fires. Be gentle with yourself and to those around you. Perhaps dance a little, or move in some way you don't normally move. You might be surprised to find that your awareness melts into her graceful movement in you.

18) Kṛśānuḥ (She Who Is Fire, the Female Deity of Fire)

You are the female deity of fire, Kṛśānuḥ, and the source of this fire is your own wisdom. In fact, your own desire and yearning for union are what fan the flames. You are benevolent. You aren't burning up others; you are igniting your own wisdom bliss and using it to burn off all that keeps you separate. This is the fire of transformation, and you are the crucible. Your yoni and generative organs are the crucible. There are gifts here. This is love. This is the source of your own self-love, and the source of love moving into the world. What if you knew this? Knew that your womb was the site of this bliss-love? Knew that your womb was the center of your body?

This fire, her fire, your fire, is more like a warming hearth fire that nourishes and sustains rather than a burning-down-the-house kind of energy. Can you bring your awareness to it as a stable, supportive, glowing ember in the center of your belly? This is the ongoing fire that we bank at night to keep our homes warm, and then fan in the morning to reawaken. This is the small drop of blazing fire that is in the center of your pelvis, the drop of liquid firelight at the core of the yoniverse. Can you sense this fire in your inner world, the tiny pinprick of heat in the bindu of your yoni-womb? It's a little below the navel, a couple of inches, and inside. Observe the movement of hot energies that are the fire drop in this bindu. It's right there, even if hidden or quiet. It's the truth of who you are, and can't be damaged by any life circumstances, or events, or wounding. Our true nature cannot be tarnished or blemished or diminished by life. Our true nature is ultimate reality, and thus our true nature is primordial: ādyā. It's always there, perfect, whole, waiting for you to feel again, and use to find your way home.

Take some time today to put your own loving healing hands on your pelvis, and let this circuitry run. Sense how the energies move. Breathe into your womb and hands and let them move the sacred energies of fire. This is the work of Kṛśānuh-Kālī. Your hands as her hands. Your pelvis as hers. Your fire and her fire as the one fire. Feel this fire, yoginīs and yogis.

19) Kapilā (She Who Is the Tawny-Colored One)

Tawny? I was a bit confused at first by this simple reference to Kapilā being a color that is not usually associated with any of Kālī's forms. And then I went back in the liturgy to the fire of Kṛśānuḥ from yesterday, and ahead to the blackness of tomorrow's name, Kṛṣṇā. Then I understood. Of course! We are *in* her fire, cooking, not to a crisp, but to the perfection of golden tawny doneness. Kapilā is the tawniness of a doe's eye, milk chocolate in the hand, caramels in the mouth, roasted chestnuts, toasted marshmallows, golden honey dripping from the hive, ginger tea, single malt scotch in sunlight, the crust on a lovely loaf of bread just before cutting, and autumn leaves as the wind dances them.

Kapilā-Kālī is the one who remembers to take us out of the oven on time, revealing our perfection. She knows how much cooking we really need to allow this work to take place. Imagine, right here, on day nineteen of our sādhana, that you are perfectly done. This is perfection, in the mess and grit and pain and joy. Right now, in this minute, this is what golden perfection is. Your own perfection is under/through everything else that you are experiencing right now.

I looked at Wikipedia's definition of "tawny" and found a sampling of color swatches. Exciting! Do look, and pick the color of your own perfect roasting. Then, put your hands on your pelvis and imagine that your whole being is perfect, tawny, Kapilā perfection. It truly is.

20) Kṛṣṇā (She Who Is Black)

As we've been discussing, the Tantric path is that of full inclusion. Everything gets brought into her lap. In the same way, as you may already know, black is not the absence of color but contains all colors within itself. Everything included.

In your part of the web of the yoniverse, can you identify something you have been turning away from? If so, would you like to turn towards it a little more, trusting in Kṛṣṇā-Kālī's darkness, and knowing she can carry it all?

In addition, Kṛṣṇa (with the short "a") is a blue-black deity in his own right. Black meeting black here in the great love union: their black enhancing each other's primordial blackness. Can you feel how the peaceful deity meets the fierce deity in union? Both deities take on the qualities of the other, and black merges with black. Kṛṣṇa-Kṛṣṇā-Kālī inseparable.

21) Kṛṣṇānandavivarddhinī (She Who Is the Increaser of the Bliss of the Dark One, Kṛṣṇa)

Increasing Kṛṣṇa's bliss is part of Kālī's job description and the essence of her vital self. She was made to enter into union with Kṛṣṇa, to generate bliss, and then to increase it. This is the dance of the feminine and masculine energies. This is the work of the polarities in our subtle bodies, our gross bodies, in the bodies of the deities, and in the body of the cosmos. We are here to practice into union and bliss and awareness. Love is another term for bliss, most days.

Can you imagine that you embody Kṛṣṇānandavivarddhinī-Kālī and that your existence is a grace, a gift offered to the world? Your feminine embodiment increases the bliss of the entire cosmos; that's just the nature of the feminine, and the source of the true form of her embodied power, her śakti. In addition, you are not separate from the divine masculine, the black Kṛṣṇa. What joy I feel in my subtle body, right now, as I write this and feel this enlivening.

Place your hands on your body as you contemplate this name. What do you experience?

22) Kālarātriḥ (She Who Is the Night of Darkness)

In this recitation of her names, I'm feeling a movement, a flow, between the moments of union, and moments in which I remember the blessings of darkness. We are moving with these energies, back and forth, sometimes abruptly, and at other times the movement happens slowly, over the course of evoking several of these names.

Here, in the first name of a new stanza, we have moved from the increase of bliss in union with Kṛṣṇa to the texture of the night of darkness, the night-time portion of the darkness. This is the deepest darkness, the quietest hour, when nary a thing moves . . . so deep is this quiet dark. We can hear forever in this darkness, even when our sight is useless. Kālarātriḥ is this velvet night, in the moment after the bliss. At first we sigh with only ahhhs and yesess, and then the night of darkness arrives, and we experience things we don't normally experience. We are suddenly available to that which was previously unavailable to us. We let ourselves drop into that night of darkness with her, as her.

This night of darkness is extremely precious. When we let go of efforting with the eyes, and drop into all the other senses, we let go of our normal habits of relating to the world and to others, and explore a new territory. Have you ever covered your eyes and explored the world without sight, without light, for an hour or day? If you do this for any length of time, your other senses become heightened. It's a different way of relating to all that you are familiar with. So precious is this experiment that some Tantric lineages have practices that include retreats done in total darkness, with no clocks or other timekeeping. We can make friends with the dark in this way and allow ourselves to move outside the realm of normal time, relative time. The embodied wisdom of Kālarātriḥ is offering to let us melt into her night of darkness and move from the world of relative time to absolute time (truly Kālī's realm). What is Kālarātriḥ-Kālī offering you with her night of darkness? Can you taste this time-out-of-time movement, and the wisdom there is in this?

23) Kāmarūpā (She Who Is the Form of Desire)

The night of darkness moves us into the form of desire. Darkness and desire are linked here, in these names and in these practices. This is Kāmarūpā, she who is the form of desire. Kāmarūpā is also known as Kāmākhyā, who is the menstruating goddess in Assam, India. Kāmākhyā-Kāmarūpā is known as a form of Kālī. She is also known affectionately as Kāmākṣī (mother of love and desire). One of the literal translations of her name is "Renowned Goddess of Desire." As I've noted at length in the Introduction, the Kāmākhyā temple is one of my spiritual homes, and I have much to share with you about Kāmarūpā, Kāmākhyā, the goddess who is the center (the bindu) of my kula. I will repeat much of that information here to reinforce it, and give you another chance to taste of her blessings.

Kāmākhyā is the goddess of desire, the form of desire. *Kāma* is the Sanskrit term for "desire," the root word of her name. Kāmākhyā is full blown sexual desire. As we have touched on elsewhere, in this tradition we bring desire onto the spiritual path.

Kāmākhyā sits in the center, in the bindu, of the temple hill in Assam, and also in the center of a larger cosmology revolving around the goddesses' scattered body parts (temples arose to house the body parts and are often referred to as Śākta Pīṭha). Kāmākhyā is surrounded by the Yoginīs, the Mātṛkās, and the Mahāvidyās. Kāmākhyā takes this central seat because she is the primordial (ādyā) goddess, the primordial yoni goddess at the premiere yoni-pīṭha.

Kālī-Kāmarūpā-Kāmākhyā is a menstruating goddess, and many of the families that live at the Kāmākhyā temple understand that the most potent manifestation of a woman's śakti is her menstrual blood. Again, as I've pointed out previously, at Kāmākhyā, menstruation is highly auspicious, full of life force, and therefore must be attended to carefully. Menstruation is the starting point of creation, and holds the vital life force of the cosmos.

Kāmākhyā is the bindu of all the Śākta Pīṭha in South Asia, around which all manifestation (and all the other body parts) swirl, ebb and flow, like great tidal forces moving and shifting in harmony with the other elemental forces. Because she is this primordial elemental energy, Kāmākhyā has no form (rūpā) and no mūrti (statue) in which her divine presence has been installed, as is common in most other Hindu temples. Instead, she is her yoni, desire itself. She is a cleft in the bedrock from which a spring emerges. Here Kāmākhyā is Kāmarūpā: the form of desire.

In your own life, can you feel the relationship between menstruation and desire, between the movement of śakti and the movement of desire? What would it be like to transmute "desire" into "Desire" and "union" into "Union"? What role might the night of darkness have in this? What role might Kāmarūpā play in this? What role might you play in this?

24) Kāmapāśavimocinī (She Who Is the Liberator from the Bonds of Desire)

I love this aspect of Kālī: she brings desire, is the form of desire, and also liberates us from any bonds/shackles/afflictions that may have attached themselves to that desire. She brings it and removes it. Oh, the paradoxical Tantric mysteries continue to unfold and reveal themselves.

As you continue to open towards the expression of your desire, do you experience any stickiness or shadow aspects there? Is there wounding that has somehow twisted desire? If so, make extra prayers and offerings to Kāmapāśavimocinī-Kālī, asking to be freed from these woundings and shadow aspects. Gently bring yourself to Kāmapāśavimocinī and ask to be freed. As you lay your hands on your body in front of your Kālī shrine, what happens once you are free?

25) Kādambinī (She Who Is as Dark as a Bank of Rainclouds)

She is dark, as we have been experiencing in the past three weeks. Darker than dark, the darkest dark. Velvet dark night without stars. What Kādambinī brings to this experience is that this darkness is neither still nor static. Instead, Kādambinī-Kālī shows us the elemental forces inherent in the darkness. This is the alive darkness that will burst into a thunderstorm at any moment. Notice how the air becomes a little more charged and alive just before the thunder crackles? Notice how vibrant it all is before the rain actually falls? There is so much that is unknown in those moments; we don't know how much rain will fall, nor in what direction. Will it be soft and gentle, or crazy wild, whipping our hair and clothing almost to shreds? Will we be nourished? Excited? Terrified? Or perhaps excitedly nourishingly terrified? This is Kādambinī bringing the pulsating, dark, elemental energies that emerge from the dark.

This is some crazy life we are living, isn't it? Some amazing sādhana we are doing! Relish this vibrancy that is quivering in the unknown dark space before the elements unfurl. This is the primordial bindu. Can you stay present with her vibrancy, her unpredictable aliveness? How about your own? What of your vibrancy and unpredictable feminine aliveness? Can you bear it? Let yourself drink it in with a knowing smile. This is your bindu as well.

26) Kalādhārā (She Who Is the Bearer of the Crescent Moon and All Female Energy)

Kalādhārā is the form of Kālī that holds all the feminine energies that comprise the primordial matrix of existence. She is the storehouse of all śakti. As such, in this description, Kalādhārā-Kālī is the one who bears, carries, or wears, the crescent moon. Like other names we have already encountered, we see here how Kālī actually holds the primordial śakti matrix of the energies that are normally associated with the gods. The crescent moon is usually a sign that Śiva is present. Kalādhārā reminds us that it is she who is bearing Śiva. Once he has manifested, they then switch roles, and he holds her up so she can continue to dance. There is a saying that goes something like, "Without Kālī, Śiva is just a corpse." She animates him, then he offers her the support and structure necessary for her dance to continue. It's a beautiful interweaving of energies here.

To be able to be present for the depth and richness of this intermingled dance of union, we have to first come to terms with our own womb-yoni-pelvic-matrix. Kalādhārā asks us to feel into our own female energies, our own śakti, especially as it manifests in the womb-yoni-pelvis, the center of our bodies. Do you sense the energies moving there? Can you feel how the pelvis is the source of existence, the birthing of all that we know, as well as the same energy that births the cosmos? Is there any aspect of your own pelvic-womb energies that you have quieted or turned away from? Is any part wounded? If so, please take today as an opportunity to work with this. You might even want to dedicate your recitation of her names to the healing and activation of your own womb-pelvis, and the womb of all existence.

27) Kalikalmaṣanāśinī (She Who Is the Destructress of Evil in the Dark Age of Kālī)

Kālī's fiercest aspects come forth here in Kalīkalmaṣanāśinī: She destroys evil in the most dark times. What I love about this is that Kalikalmaṣanāśinī's fierceness is used for our benefit; all her scary aspects, intense qualities, fierce energies, and frightening ways are actually being used to relieve our suffering.

Bringing Kalikalmaṣanāśinī into your awareness with love and gratitude, can you feel how something fierce or frightening in your experience might actually be a blessing? How might her capacity to destroy evil, even when wearing such a fierce aspect, be for your benefit?

Use this face of Kālī, as Kalikalmaṣanāśinī, to support you in moving towards what you are afraid of with more openness and love. She's got your back, you know? And your front. Every bit of you is under her care. It just might not look like what you expect at first.

28) Kumārīpūjanaprītā (She Who Loves the Worship of the Virgin-Girls)

I love the worship of the *Kumārī,** the virgin girls who are understood to be embodiments of Devī. As devotees and practitioners, we work with Kālī in both outer and inner forms as a practice of union; we work to understand that we are not separate from all that arises as reality, and that the outer world is an integral part of the cakra that is all reality. We work with the practices of inner and outer mirroring in a variety of ways. We go on pilgrimage, for example, to come into contact with external forms of Devī that are truly our own inner forms coming to life in the presence of her. We practice sādhana. We do pūjā, ritual. We work to see all beings as divine, as deities actually.

This is also why, in the Kālīkula, we worship women as goddess, as Devī. Our active worship of women as goddess reinforces this worldview, this understanding of the way our ordinary lives are extensions of the mysterious work of the cosmos, the cakra of ultimate reality. We worship women in refined esoteric rituals as well as in daily life with no special parameters or ritual forms. We do all this, on so many levels and in so many ways, to remember over and over again that we are part of the mystery, and that the mystery is dancing us, as Kālī, with every breath.

We worship women in all stages of the life-cycle: young pre-menstrual virgin girls, married women, and even widows. Each age of our life has its own divine form. Kumārīpūjanaprītā is the form of Kālī that understands the sanctity of the worship of the Kumārī, the virgin girls. Having participated in many Kumārī Pūjās as well as having studied it as a cultural phenomenon, I have seen these young women embrace their own self-worth as a result of this worship, awe, and respect.

The adoration of the Kumārī is not restricted to ritual settings, but extends to daily life as well. At the Kāmākhyā temple in Assam, these Kumārī truly are free, alive, and well loved. As one shopkeeper explained to me after a troupe of Kumārī walked off with the sweets in his candy jars, "When the girls are pleased, Devī is pleased." Pleasing goddess by pleasing women is a common theme at Kāmākhyā.

I hope you can go back and revision your own childhood right now. As that bumper sticker says, "It's never too late to have a happy childhood." Revision yours so that you know you were well loved, well pleased, and respected. Imagine wild freedom combined with community adoration. Imagine knowing that you were the goddess. Imagine this for all your daughters now too. What might change were this so? Even if it's not possible in your circumstances to offer all this to your own daughters, can you choose a worldview for yourself that allows this to be so? Feel all of us in Kumārīpūjanaprītā's care of the Kumārī, of yourself as a Kumārī, as your daughter-Kumārī. How might your world change as a result of this love of the virgin-girls?

29) Kumārīpūjakālayā (She Who Is the Refuge of all Virgin Worshippers)

Kālī loves the worship of the Kumārī, the pre-menarchal girls, that we enact Kālī's love through Kumārī Pūjā. This precious form of worship allows us to integrate an internal understanding of all women, all beings actually, as manifestations of the divine. We know these gorgeous girls as goddess, in girl form. We don't get too fixated on any one girl: this is not about a single special girl, at least not in India and Nepal, but that every girl is this special. Then she grows up and moves into other forms of Devī, other forms of embodying Mā. All of us go through these cycles in our life, and Kālī is right there with us at every stage. No part of us is unrevered.

Those of us who participate in this worldview—those who undertake this darśan of the Kumārī—are held in Kumārīpūjakālayā's love. For those of us who practice seeing Kālī in all women, and especially in these girls, Kumārīpūjakālayā is our refuge, our sanctuary. Kumārīpūjakālayā-Kālī says:

> Come rest your weary body here. This is hard work we are doing. Rest here. I am your sanctuary. I am the well you drink from. I am the round tent where you gather with the others, near the river, with a fire pit, for several days of rest. Come here, let yourself take a break from the rigors of life and find the softness in your own body. Let's sing a soft body-love song together. I'm here to protect you. I'm here to nourish you. Healing is here with me. Know all women as Devī, no matter how they act, no matter what they believe, no matter what they do. Know all women as such, yourself included. I'm here to support you in that view, in meeting that reality without obstruction. I'm here to let you feel this directly in your own body.

What an exquisite blessing to come home to this refuge that Kumārīpūjakālayā offers.

30) Kumārībhojanānandā (She Who Is Completely Joyed by the Feasts and Gifts to the Virgin-Girls)

Not only does Kālī love the worship of Kumārī, she is pleased with the sacred feasts and gifts to the Kumārī that go along with Kumārī Pūjā. These feasts and giftings are part of most of the extended rituals of the Kālīkula, and are quite a sensual delight. Kumārībhojanānandā reminds us to put out offerings on the shrine and eat in a sacred way. These small actions can be daily reminders of our connection with Kālī, and are part of the development of our relationship with Kālī, just as they are part of relationship building with most people. Eat together, share time, exchange energies and gifts. At the next holiday that you spend with family and friends, perhaps you might consider how feasting and sharing time with loved ones is a ritual feast? Can you see Devī in everyone at the table? Can you see the food as sacrament? Can you feel the web matrix of union glistening in the room? Kumārībhojanānandā-Kālī reminds us that, anytime we gather with loved ones and share food or gifts, we are in sacred space. It pleases her. Perhaps spend extra time with a Kumārī in your world in the next days, and see if you can please her too.

31) Kumārīrūpadhāriṇī (She Who Is Herself in the Form of a Virgin-Girl)

Through all of the ways that Kālī is pleased by the worship of the Kumārī, in the end, here at the last name in this stanza, we discover that Kālī is actually a Kumārī herself. She has taken the form of Kumārī, and thus is Kumārīrūpadhāriṇī.

This way that Kālī has of first appearing separate from something, loving it fully, protecting it, and then merging into it indivisibly, is Kālī's way and one of her most central teachings. Can you intuit in your own body wisdom, and feel from your womb-yoni, how Kālī can love the worship of Kumārī, be the refuge for Kumārī worshippers, be pleased by or with gifts and feasts to the Kumārī, and also be the form of Kumārī, all at the same time? Play with putting on your Kālī-tinted glasses and merging with this microcosmic-macrocosmic worldview. You are inseparable from all aspects of the Kumārī and their worship, as Kālī comes at union from all angles, leaving nothing/no one aside.

Extending this view out in the other direction, can Kumārīrūpadhāriṇī be separate from the Kālī of the cremation grounds?

With these last few names, I have been remembering all the Kumārī whom I have worshipped, and the Kumārī who are currently in my life. I've been more aware of the Kumārī in my neighborhood as I walk down the street or enter a shop. I also wonder about myself, when I was a Kumārī. Given Kālī's nature as a healer and as divine mother, this might be a good moment to reflect back on your Kumārī self. Is there anything from that time of your life that is unhealed and needs attention? Is there any wounding there that continues to be with you now, even though you are in a different stage of life? Perhaps you can journal about anything unhealed, and then offer that wounding up to Kumārīrūpadhāriṇī, asking for healing and transformation. Ask her to let all the parts of your Kumārī-self be whole and healed and beautiful. Do this so that you can be fully present today, as a whole being—full, mature, healed. Do this for yourself and the women in your life. Do this work in the past so you can arrive here, today, fully embodied, fierce, empowered, and know yourself as Kumārīrūpadhāriṇī.

32) Kadambavanasañcārā (She Who Is a Wanderer [Gopī] in the Kadamba Forest)

Reciting this name offers no easy transition, beloveds. How did we get from being a Kumārī to being a *Gopī,** from being a pre-menarchal, adored girl-goddess to being a mature woman living in the forest of desire, waiting for Kṛṣṇa or Pārvatī to come back? This transition takes courage and some fierceness to move through.

Self-care is vital right here. Perhaps drink some warm water and breathe deeply just now. Thank goddess at least we got a stanza break in which to pause and breathe fully before moving on to this name. Thank goddess for the wisdom inherent in the format and structure of this liturgy. Thank Devī, these names have wisdom that emerges as support and structure as we go in even more deeply. I need more chai right now. I'm making shrine offerings and lighting candles. It's that kind of moment.

Inhale. Exhale. Pause. Inhale. Exhale. Pause. Inhale. Exhale. Pause. Remember that all the names are weaving together. A piece of the matrix is forming. A glimpse of the pattern can be seen. This is the glimpse into the world of full-blown union. It's staggeringly beautiful, and so immense that it can knock us off our feet, or send us off into crazy land. I'd like to invite you to sit quietly for a moment. Can you re-member yourself? Perhaps you can extend your attention out into the world and touch the energies of the others who are also practicing the *Song of the Hundred Names of Ādyā Kālī*. Pull inwards towards yourself and simultaneously energetically lean into the other practitioners. We can trust the circle to hold us as we see more of the path unfold. Inhale. Exhale. Pause. Inhale. Exhale. Pause. Inhale. Exhale. Pause.

Who is Kadambavanasañcārā? Let's remember some of the earlier names. Do you recall Kālī's relationship to Kṛṣṇa in the twentieth and twenty-first names, Kṛṣṇā and Kṛṣṇānanda-vivarddhinī? We are picking up those threads and weaving them in here. Have you already noticed that Kālī is one of the Gopī, a woman whose practice of union is a grand love affair with Kṛṣṇa?

As we practice into union, we begin to fill with desire. Yet, even the yoginīs who are overflowing, brimming over, dripping with desire, aren't in physical union every moment of every day. Still, they are in union. That's the state that the wandering yoginīs reached, women whose lives are examples to us: Mirabai, Lalla, Lalitavajra, Dakini Lion-Face, and Yid Trogma. This is where Bandhe lives with Shaza Khandro, Lopamudra,

Lakshminkara and Lilavajra. Cudala and Shakya Devī are here, together with the old hag.[1] This is the path of the householder and the celibate. The mother, the nun, the sacred prostitute, and the temple dancer. What these women practitioners, accomplished yoginīs, share with us—no matter whether there is a living embodied beloved or consort, or whether the consort is the divine itself—is that walking in union, walking with union, is the only way to go.

If we can trust the written life stories and oral histories of these women, when we look into their worlds we see that this path isn't about being with our beloved or consort sexually every day. This is the path of practicing towards union every moment, and that can include lovemaking and sexual practices as they arise. We practice embodied sexual union so that we have a glimpse of the ultimate union, and then infuse every moment of existence with that. This doesn't happen on the first try, nor overnight. There are many challenges on the path that will confront us as we hold this awareness. That's why it's called *practice*.

This understanding, that union with a physical beloved or consort ebbs and flows, has brought forth some of the most sublime divine-love poetry on the planet. When our beloved consort Kṛṣṇa-Śiva-Bhairava or Radhā-Pārvatī-Bhairavī is gone, we yearn. We wail. We pull our hair. We complain. Then, secretly, we are delighted to have time and space to ourselves. We might exhale. We take to rolling around in the riverbank mud with our sakhī. We braid our hair, henna our feet, stop cooking for a time. And after we are undone into our feminine nature with our companions, we realize that we miss our beloved. And then we start to yearn for union because they are somewhere else.

We don't know when the beloved will return to the forest of union with us, how long they will stay when they do show up, nor if they will even be with us when they get here. We let all of this undo us, take us apart. We let the yearning drop from the heart to the womb, we let it drip downwards like warm honey and butter. This is womb business, dear sakhī.

Kadambavanasañcārā is the mature female practitioner whose true home is in the forest of union, an unmarked kadamba forest at the edge of civilization. She is there, doing her practices, hanging out with the other gopī-yoginī-sakhī, taking care of her nearly feral children, and walking in full union. Practicing in full union. Even when Kṛṣṇa or Pārvatī have left the area.

If we are able to feel the warm honey-butter of union dripping down and shifting our center of gravity from the heart to the womb, and we do this with full breath and tongue resting on the palate, we might begin to feel the traces of the energetics of our subtle body open. Kadambavanasañcārā, along with all the other accomplished yoginīs that I named, is a mature female practitioner with an enlivened subtle body. The crucible of the subtle body is the pelvic region, the yoni. This is the cauldron, the skull cup, where transformation occurs, where union occurs, and desire is transformed. The heart melts because the yoni simmers. Sometimes we don't even feel the yoni crucible simmering, heating up, until we notice our heart. That's just fine, no matter what the order of the unfolding. Just remember to let the heart's energies drip down into the yoni crucible. These women live from the womb, with it on fire, ablaze with recognition, alive in relationship to *what is*. So do we.

In all of this, it is natural for yearning to arise. There is a yoga of yearning just as there is a yoga of union. The kadamba forest holds both of these yogas, and more. This is our sacred ground. This is where the finest and most intact yoginī temples still exist.

So, while the transition to this stanza is a big transition, from girl-goddess to mature female practitioner—we can do this together. The names and stanzas of the liturgy that come after Kadambavanasañcārā show us how to live in the kadamba forest, what we do there, what rituals we undertake, what are the inner processes, and what darśan/view we can hold. Kadambavanasañcārā is a rite of passage.

Perhaps you can imagine that you are with me here: I am at the edge of the kadamba forest, where the cultivated fields give way to brambles and dense trees, to viney entanglement and lush wild flowers. I am sitting at this edge, on my heels, a cup of spicy chai in my hands after a powerful dark moon. I signal for you to come this way, over here. Let me show you the doorway in. The passage may look narrow and dangerous from out there, yet I promise that there is a sublime paradise on the other side of this tangle of thickets. Bring your children, bring your cooking pot, bring some food, your practices, some offerings. Don't forget a blanket to sleep under, and something for the feminine arts of adornment. It's all sacred embodiment practice and we will do it together, wandering here and there in the kadamba forest.

33) Kadambavanavāsinī (She Who Is a Dweller in the Kadamba Forest)

Such intensity yesterday, and today; a small reminder of the paradoxes of Kālī's ways. Not only does she wander in the kadamba forest, she dwells there too. This is the homeland of those of us on the path of the yoginī. No matter where else we might be, or what we might be doing, we are actually dwelling in the kadamba forest of union with Kadambavanavāsinī-Kālī. It reminds me of a poem by Lalla, aka Lal Ded or Lalleshwari, an eighth century wandering yoginī from South Asia. Her worldview states this more perfectly than I ever could. Just know that "jasmine garden" is another way of saying "kadamba forest."

I, Lalla, entered the jasmine garden,
where Śiva and Śākti were making love.

I dissolved into them,
and what is this
to me, now?

I seem to be here,
but really I'm walking
in the jasmine garden.
(Barks 1992:42) [2]

May we always live here as Kadambavanavāsinī-Kālī, walking in the jasmine garden inside the kadamba forest. What a sublime existence!

34) Kadambapuṣpasantoṣā (She Who Takes Delight in the [Brilliant Yellow] Flowers of the Kadamba Forest)

The prevalence of the kadamba tree is what makes this sultry place we find ourselves in a magical kadamba forest. This South Asian tree has brilliant yellow (sometimes red) bisexual flowers that are lush and highly fragrant. The kadamba flower is one of the primary ingredients in attar, a perfume that has a sandalwood base and an essential oil infused in it. Attars are one of the most precious forms of perfume, and one of the most highly prized form of an essential oil.

These flowers that Kadambapuṣpasantoṣā delights in are also often used to make the garlands (mālā) that one places around the neck of one's beloved. Under this tree, separated lovers are reunited. Under this tree, surrounded by this passionate fragrance and hidden by the leafy cover, we find ourselves intertwined with the beloved, whom we thought we had lost. Indeed, intertwined here amidst these flowers, what is there but delight? Naturally, Kadambapuṣpasantoṣā-Kālī has no other purpose. It's nothing but union now.

35) Kadambapuṣpamālinī (She Who Wears a Garland of Kadamba Flowers)

So, here we are, in this lush forest of union, wearing a gorgeous garland of brilliant yellow kadamba flowers. My sakhī are down by the river, and I'm here waiting for my consort to arrive. And, as one of my sakhī reminds me, before she goes to join the others and leave us in privacy: "Oh by the way . . . just because we're in the kadamba forest, it's not happily ever after." We may be garlanded as consort with the precious kadamba flowers, ready and waiting, and it can still be really rough. What if they don't show up? What if I'm scared and they get scared? What if I frighten them off because I'm too much woman, too much wombyn, too much yoginī? What if they are passive aggressive, have a drinking problem, three other beloveds, and bad breath? What's a yoginī to do? One moment it's union, the next separation and grief. One moment is eternal and the next is despair. As my sakhī also asked: "We signed up for this?" Actually we did. And it can be awful. Which is why I'm so grateful for the practice, the sādhana, the foundation that shows me how to hold this all, how to be in the room—pissy as hell, but in the room—and watching the room at the same time. Breathing it all through, letting the womb take the edge off it. Staying seated on my tiger skin seat. You can't dislodge me that easily! I get to stay in union, on my seat/āsana, no matter what. We cultivate this incredible view, and then we have ample opportunities to practice this view.

I have this moment of challenge as Kadambapuṣpamālinī, wearing the flower garland of consortship, in order to remember that taking my seat, as a mature yoginī, as a mature woman, is not dependent on what other people think of me, nor how they react to me (assuming that I'm acting maturely, wisely, and with as much grace and kindness as I can). It is also not dependent on external conditions, nor is it dependent on the other person.

Kadambapuṣpamālinī takes her seat as consort in union no matter the outer circumstances. She has earned the right to wear the kadamba flower mālā because of the depth of her practice, and because she has taken her seat as a mature yoginī. This is what we practice towards, and this is what we practice for.

The next stanzas in this liturgy tell us that not only is there the sweet delight of full blown life and love in the kadamba forest, there is also the reminder of change, death, decay, and transformation. The sweetness has a taste of the fierce, and the fierceness will have a taste of the sweet. It's all mixed up together and we have to be able to take all the flavors of union in, to turn *towards* all the flavors. Otherwise, it's not union. Remind yourself of the beauty in the midst of suffering, and the grace of suffering in the midst of beauty.

No matter the flavor of the day, there is nowhere else I'd rather be. Especially since I get to be here with all of you.

36) Kiśorī (She Who Is Ever Youthful)

Here with Kiśorī, we come back from teetering on the edge of "all-pissy-consort-disaster" to resting in the fresh blossoming of love in the heart-womb. From new and fresh to old and jaded to eternally young. We have it all here in the kadamba forest with Kālī. The experience that we are sharing in the forest is a chaotic ride—like being on a roller coaster that twists and turns through the spiral of the feminine matrix. As we ride, we sense flavor after flavor of love present in the feminine form. Today's name is a reminder to not hold any moment too tightly, as it will change, probably soon, just as the beauty of youth can change with no warning. One moment we are a Kumārī, the next we are in the midst of mature yoginī consort practice, and then, whoooosh, right back to Kiśorī, ever youthful.

Kiśorī also asks us to give up our fixed notions of time and space. Kālī the hag-crone who is as ancient as the cosmos is young and ever youthful simultaneously. What is it like to hold both truths in your body simultaneously? Might Kālī-Kiśorī be pointing us towards a timeless time and a spaceless space? In this womb-matrix of existence that are we in, time stops and starts at her will. Space exists and ceases existing at her whim. Can you step into this worldview even when it appears that the calendars will continue endlessly? What if the world doesn't end? What if there is no apocalypse, ever? Kiśorī shows us that it keeps going. The world will end and be always fresh too. She is always birthing the cosmos into manifestation, that's Kiśorī. And, that's us too. Every inhale is this birthing. Every holding/retention of the breath, in the soft middle space, is the preservation. Every exhale is the transformation/dissolution. Feel that entire cycle in your body/being. Let Kiśorī lead you in here, to this exploration. Hold your tongue to your palate as you do so and let your belly be full. Discover the womb-cosmos-matrix in your own belly. Know yourself as Kiśorī on the inhale.

37) Kalakaṇṭhā (She Who Has a Soft and Deep-Throated Voice [That Resounds with the Transformative Mantra])

Kalakaṇṭhā takes us right back into the mystery of life and death, beauty and bloodshed, all wrapped up together. What does it take to transform suffering, loss, and horror into pleasure, love, and life? Kalakaṇṭhā-Kālī's soft and deep-throated voice is the sound of a Billie Holiday singing "Strange Fruit": it is sultry, passionate, and fully available for the ravages of life's horror-mysteries. Lady Day (as Billie Holiday is sometimes known), and others, use their voices to tap on the crusty parts of our interiors and exteriors. Kalakaṇṭhā-Kālī says, "Let this in. Drink here, so you know what is true. We can do something about this, if we let it in." Because, dear beloveds, that which we can let in, imbibe, not armor against, is that which we have the capacity to transform. If it remains outside us, the transformational alchemy of Tantra does not occur. We have to drink it all in, bringing it down into the cauldron of the womb-yoni-pelvis. When we have drunk it, tasted it, swallowed it, eaten it, we can actually address suffering and transform it.

Let Kalakaṇṭhā's voice be the sultry love song that awakens you to your truest embodied wisdom. If you were going to sing a love song of awakening, so fierce that it resounds as a transformative mantra, what is the name of that song you would sing? What is the tone, rhythm, scale, duration? Are there lyrics? Today, with your soft hand touching your throat, write the soft-bodied love song that allows something you are pushing away, holding at arm's length, to trickle into your being. Allow in that which you have been armored against. Let it in. Drip it down into your belly using your breath (with tongue on palate), and place your hands on your body as encouragement. Once it is in your belly, feel it. Truly feel the whole thing. Rage, cry, deny, shout, grieve, do that angry shake-em-down dance, break dishes, throw lamps. Now, with your womb-yoni-pelvis as the cauldron, you are ready to transform it. Resting into your meditation seat in front of your Kālī shrine, use your mantra, or the recitation of these names, as the fierce transformative mantra that creates honey out of poison. Use your transformative mantra and these names to transform the pain/suffering/agony/closure. What is this process like for you? What emerges, what is left, what ambrosia or amṛta do you encounter along the way?

38) Kalanādaninādinī (She Who Is Sweet as the Cakravāka Bird)

Transformative mantras dripping with honey-song yesterday, and then sweet honey-song back in the kadamba forest today (with a taste of bitterness, of course). Truly I revel in what amazing training this is. It moves fast, and provides us with the capacity and fluidity for navigating our daily lives, and for opening to our own awakening.

The cakravāka is a South Asian bird that looks like a golden duck with a black beak, the tips of the tail feathers are also dipped in black. Kapilā meets Kālī here. They are also called "Brahminy ducks."

The cakravāka is known for binding itself to its beloved in union, even when apart. A kind of faithfulness to union, to the beloved, allows this sweetness. At night, their voices move out across the waters, as they sweetly call to their own beloveds to return, to reunite for evening love play. Kalanādaninādinī shows us how our longing and yearning for union, and nightly re-union, are the sweetness of consort practice at play. Tonight . . . will she/he come? Is that her/his voice I hear on the other side of this marsh? Let me call out to discover the mutual recognition of our union. This is the sweetness of amṛta flowing, nectar moving. This is the sweetness of knowing the beloved even when separated. Given that the cakravāka engages in love play all year long, no matter the season or weather, we see the endless possibilities of līlā that are not dependent on the outer circumstances. This is the sweetness of union, no matter what. And the bittersweetness of the yoga of yearning when apart.

Cakravāka birds are also associated with the feminine arts of adornment. Our adornment is a way to come into embodiment more fully, to mark our embodiment, to draw us back into our bodies. We can nourish our bodies through adornment, and remember who we are as well. There are practices around wearing specific forms of adornment in order to train the body, support body opening, prepare the body for union practices.

Sweetness of union is tangible. I can taste Kalanādaninādinī in my mouth. I can feel her warmth and blessings moving down my body, opening my subtle channels, breathing moisture into the closed and dry places. What a blessing she is today, to me, to us.

May Kalanādaninādinī's sweetness be with you today.

39) Kādambarīpānaratā (She Who Drinks the Wine-Nectar of the Kadamba Fruit)

The moon is often at play when I undertake my evening practices. Last night, I drank her wine nectar as I practiced. Kādambarīpānaratā is drinking the sweet nectar that flows from the practices of union. In this lineage, and in these teachings, *wine-nectar* can refer to many things. It's part of the Tantric twilight language. On the outer levels, of course, it refers to the distilled spirits that one can make from the nectar of the kadamba fruit.

Brewing and distilling spirits are one of the metaphors for the alchemical transformation of Tantric practices. One finds a reliable recipe, gathers the ingredients, prepares the ingredients, sets up the distilling process, and during the brewing, something happens. Things change. Alchemy is afoot. At the end, there is an enchanting liquor, a wine-nectar, a tangible outcome. This mirrors our practice and is one of the reasons that historically so many yoginīs and yogins were wine makers, beer brewers, and distillers. Intoxication with spirits is one of the metaphors for union. We are so suffused with our love of Kālī, of the divine, of our beloved, of union, that we are drunk on her love, their love. From many sacred traditions there are beautiful poems about being drunk on love!

Moving inwards, uncovering other layers of meaning, wine-nectar also can refer to our own fluids. As we intensify in our practices, as they move into us on a cellular level, our blood, bone, and body fluids become imbued with the fruit of our practice. The Tantric texts and teachers indicate that we wear our practice on/in our body so tangibly that other people can literally taste it on us;

others can perceive the distinct energies of our spiritual practices. When our practice has so deeply saturated us that this happens, that it drips out of our pores as sweat, can be tasted in our tears, is part of the smell of our skin, runs in our salivary glands, and flows in our sexual fluids, we know we have gotten somewhere. It is also in highly concentrated forms in our moon blood. These levels of meaning are more than enough to intoxicate us with Kālī's love and blessings today. They are enough to intoxicate us with the beauty of our lives, with the blessings of love, with the full grace of existence. Let the wine-nectar of union flow.

❁ ❁ ❁

When we first undertook the practice of the *Song of the Hundred Names of Ādyā Kālī* as a community, at this point in the sādhana I went into silent private retreat. Spiritual retreat is a time when we turn our focus from external stimulation, withdrawing from the external world so that we can come into more connection with the inner worlds, the sacred worlds, Kālī's cosmologies, the yoniverse. We go quietly, taking time and space to dive down, through, and into the womb of her existence. Later, when we emerge, we then try to integrate this mysterious dive we have taken into the secret realms with our lives in the external, more public, realms. We bring up the treasures and pray for their manifestation as wisdom in our lives.

Retreat allows long practice sessions, study, rest, movement (yoga/dance/walk), and pleasure. Each day can include all of these elements. These are not necessarily the traditional elements of retreat (pleasure, for example, is not on any list nor in any teaching that I know of), but over the years, I have discovered that this is what works best for me, a female practitioner, to shepherd myself into the more subtle realms. While there is some structure to my days, it is not a rigid retreat schedule. This is a feminine retreat meant to support my relationship to Kālī, to these practices, and to my offerings in the world. These are the elements that support me dropping into more openness, while keeping me present for the discipline of practice.

Most people I know take retreat by going somewhere else, leaving their daily life. I don't go anywhere for retreat; instead I withdraw into my home, my personal temple and yoni crucible. I have everything I need here already and I do not need to leave home to find space to go deeply. I stock up on food, cover the mirrors so I turn inward, soften the judgments, and find my way without the external reflections. During this retreat, my bathroom mirror had a beautiful yoni goddess maṇḍala covering it so I could remember my truest face as I brushed my teeth and used my neti pot.

At times, going on retreat at retreat centers or other locales has been useful. I even took this so far that I once lived and worked at a retreat center. Yet now, I am living in the world more fully, and it serves me more to pay attention to what is emerging right here, to more firmly ground the yoni crucible that is my personal shrine and home. It takes far less effort than traveling, and is far less expensive, far less work, and far less disruption of the practice space I've developed in my own home.

❁ ❁ ❁

Drink in the blessings of practice like the sweet nectar-wine that it is. This is the grace of Mā. We are in it, bathing in it, partaking of it, drenched in our own nectar.

40) Kādambarīpriyā (She Who Is Excited and Pleased with the Kadamba Fruit Wine)

Oh this nectar is sweet and sublime. Flowing from Kālī's lips into my body, dripping down down down. There are extra offerings out this morning, on my altar, including meat and wine, as a sheer act of gratitude for the shape of this life. I am aware of how fleeting this moment is, of how insanely precious it is in the entire fabric of my life. The shape of my body/being is pressed into existence as a feminine offering. Joy. Sublime pleasure. Gratitude.

Kādambarīpriyā is my honored guest in the yoni crucible. We are sitting at the shrine passing the kadamba fruit wine back and forth slowly, speaking of the warm full taste, rich amber honey with notes of summer song and dark hollows. There is a bit of juniper berry and pear too. We notice together how it becomes pomegranate molasses when we finally swallow it. Channels opening, softening as it moves down the trunk of our bodies. We bring our breath fully into our soft bellies. Tongue on the palate. Slight whisper of awareness on the perineum. Yoni full and soft, inside and out. Kādambarīpriyā is delighted that when she sips the wine through her full mouth, that it drips out of her body at the base in the form of sexual arousal. The blazing in the belly is arising, and we are both warm, so warm.

What pleasure this is, what delight! The excitement arrives just as the mild intoxication begins to arrive. Everything softens more, and a soft cry of delight is on our lips. The beloved is here. She is right here with us. With you. Not ever separate. Can you take your seat here, in this lap, with your legs wrapped around the beloved's hips, anklets tinkling softly as you hook one foot around the other. Wrap your arms around their neck. Gaze into their eyes, left eye to left eye, with this kadamba fruit wine emboldening you, filling you, arousing you, enlivening you. Spread this love through your body and entire being with your breath. Let it fill you. Satisfy you. Nourish you. Nurture you. Transform you. Let your inhale fan the flame in the belly. Let the exhale send the love and consciousness, bliss and awareness, out into the world. Spread it around as blessing force, as love-prana, as śakti-goodness for all creation.

41) Kapālapātraniratā (She Who Is Drinking from a Skull Cup)

One stanza ends in our intoxicated enjoyment of amṛta, and the next stanza begins letting us know that we are imbibing that amṛta-nectar from a sacred vessel, a skull cup (*kapāla**).

In Tantric traditions, kapāla are sacred containers that are a reminder of how close death is, how fragile life is. The nectar may be flowing from our union, and at the same time life is short and precious. How close is death? It's as close as life. Accept death, and an embodied life is possible. Drink amṛta from this cup, and know some of the inner mysteries.

Kapālapātraniratā offers us a way through our fear of mortality and through our fear of death. Let the nectar be the guide and then the preciousness of life will emerge. One of Kālī's specialties, and we see it here in this stanza, is this ability to fully embrace death, overcome our fears, and to wear death as an ornament, an adornment, in the midst of union. She shows us how to bring it close so we are able to make friends with it. Accept death fully and we then know life. Drink this in so that we can know how real and precious embodiment is.

My own sacred space is a testament to this worldview: bones mixed in with flowers and incense. I have sacrums, vertebrae, bone ritual implements, bone adornment, and even a kapāla. The kapāla holds the space, just like the pelvic bowl, for the Tantric mysteries and transformations to take place and stabilize.

Perhaps you would like to consider adding something to your Kālī shrine today, something for death and transformation, something to acknowledge your willingness to have your fear drop away and your acceptance of death as one of the three sides of Kālī's triangle of union (birth/generation, sustenance/perseverance, transformation/death). This is Kālī's yoni, and ours too. These three aspects are, if you remember back to her first three names, the bīja of *hrīṃ*, *śrīṃ*, and *krīṃ*. Each bīja, each aspect, inseparable from the whole. This is Kālī's teaching. Look to the last names as well: this entire sādhana is sandwiched in between these three bīja. Can you drink this in, like honey wine, from a skull cup?

42) Kaṅkālamālyadhāriṇī (She Who Is Wearing a Garland of Bones)

Kaṅkālamālyadhāriṇī is the close sister of Kapālapātraniratā. Perhaps they are the same sister? As I shared a little yesterday, bringing in an awareness of the full cycle of creation/preservation/transformation is a part of Kālī's work. Wearing bone ornaments, a garland of bones, is akin to saying that we not only accept the birth/creation and preservation/sustaining aspects of Kālī's yoni but we also accept her as death/transformation/change. I wear transformation as an ornament, keeping it close to my skin. Yoginīs, ḍākinīs, and deities in the Tantric lineages often wear bone ornaments as markers of having attained inner qualities, as well as having embraced the dance of life and death as a single form of union.

Kaṅkālamālyadhāriṇī tells the story of Kālī's bone ornaments, which she wears in the cremation grounds when covered with ashes from funeral pyres. This bone mālā, garland, moves and bumps against her body as she dances life and death and preservation into a seamless whole. She says, "I am here with you in life (wearing a garland of jasmine and hibiscus), and I shall be with you in death (wearing my bone ornaments). Remember this and let your fear be eased." Indeed, one of Kālī's uplifted hands is always in the *abhaya mudrā:** fear not. This is to be celebrated, and it is why we dance, wearing her bone ornaments as a garland.

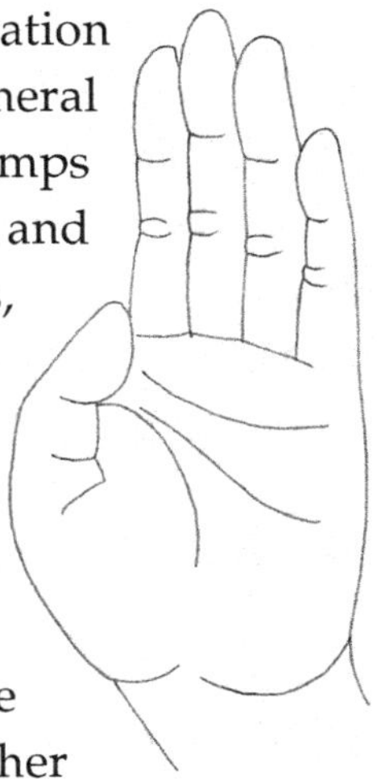

43) Kamalāsanasantuṣṭā (She Who Is a Lover of the Lotus Flower)

The beauty in these nights, as we proceed with this liturgy, may bring love so close and tangible that it presses in on us, perhaps even in our dreams. The stillness of the night may potentiate the taste of nectar/love/quiet storm/joy that may allow us to move into more subtle realms.

This form of nourishment, they say in the Tantric traditions, is what feeds us, preparing us for the full blown union. This union is understood to be the flowering of the lotus, the opening and revealing of our innermost true nature, our awakening. Kamalāsanasantuṣṭā loves the lotus flower, and she loves our awakening. Like Tārā in the Buddhist tradition, Kamalāsanasantuṣṭā is committed to our awakening in this lifetime in our female form. Use this body, she says. This is the temple. Practice, deepen, stabilize, realize, offer.

The lotus flower is also a way of describing the flowering of the yoni in desire and pleasure. What might it be like to be so fully embodied and alive that our yoni blossoms open as a lotus flower? What might it be like to be practicing so fully that our yoni amṛta-nectar is transformed into the nectar of the lotus? As Kamalāsanasantuṣṭā, what would it be like to love this lotus flower? This is Kālī's specialty: loving the yoni-lotus in each of us, as her. Can you find it in yourself to love your own yoni (the womb and the outer petals) as Kālī-Kamalāsanasantuṣṭā? Can you love your own yoni-lotus so much that it becomes the gateway to your own awakening?

44) Kamalāsanavāsinī (She Who Is Delighted to Be Seated Within the Lotus)

She is a lover of the lotus, and now she is seated within the lotus. Kālī does this wondrous dance in which she loves an item and then becomes the item. The same movement occurs for us in our own practice: we love Kālī, and then in the blink of an eye (the pulse of the womb) we are Kālī. Oh Kamalāsanavāsinī, what delight this is! There is no hassle, no drama, no drag. We just smoothly move from being ourselves in love to being love. This is sublime joy, and one of the gifts she offers us. Simple. True. Real. Alive. Union. Right here.

Kamalāsanavāsinī-Kālī also sits within the lotus, with great delight. Her āsana, seat, throne, is in the center of the lotus. We can imagine that this lotus is above our heads, in the classical cakra system, in the traditional renditions of how the subtle body blossoms in awakening. From the women's point of view inside the Kālīkula, however, there is another version of that, which no one says and everyone knows: that your cervix is also a lotus. What if Kamalāsanavāsinī-Kālī had her most primordial throne-āsana in the pelvis? Can you feel her there? What might this mean for union? Can you feel her/your delight at this? Here is the primordial matrix of all existence, the primordial womb. In her. In you. As her. As you. Delight. Joy. Bliss. Longing for union. It all arises from here.

45) Kamalālayamadhyasthā (She Who Is Abiding in the Middle of the Lotus)

Kālī not only sits in the lotus, but as Kamalālayamadhyasthā we are shown even more specificity. From outer forms to inner forms, we travel more and more inward to where she lives in the middle of the lotus. This is her natural resting place and home. Kālī-Kamalālayamadhyasthā lives in the bindu of the lotus within the lotus: the womb-lotus. This is not a temporary visit for her, this is home, the place she never strays from. This is her sanctuary. Are you able to find this knowing in your body? Could you come home to this?

If we undergo the micro-macro exchange, you are Kālī-Kamalālayamadhyasthā living in the middle of a lotus. Imagine that—your seat at your Kālī shrine is the os of her cervix, and you are therefore living in her yoni-womb. How does that affect you?

Rest your hands on your yoni-womb-pelvis and notice what you feel. Perhaps you can do the daily recitation of her names today with your hands on your yoni-womb-pelvis. What arises as you honor yourself as living in the lotus, being the lotus, and encompassing this lotus?

46) Kamalāmodamodinī (She Who Is Pleased and Intoxicated by the Scent of the Lotus)

We are sitting in, residing, dwelling within this incredible flowering yoni-lotus of nectarine embodied aliveness. As I settle in here, as Kamalāmodamodinī, I begin to notice that not only is there a soft seat here, luscious and comfortable, but also that other sensory delights begin to move into my awareness. Kamalāmodamodinī is sitting across from me, on her own lotus-seat. As I notice the tenderness of my yoni pressing into the tenderness of my lotus seat, I am also delighted to begin to notice the way the lotus smells. It has its own unique smell, as every yoni-lotus does. I discover that I like it. A lot. I fill my belly with breath, and thus with śakti-prāṇa, and I notice the impact that drinking in this scent has on my subtle body. I feel the channels soften and the bulb at the base of my body flutter. I feel my body soften and become more aware. I notice an earthiness and a simultaneous high note. I feel grounded and expanding upwards simultaneously. As Kamalāmodamodinī and I sit here more, I notice my cervix too. And a fluttering on the front wall of my uterus. I notice the anklets on my feet, their weight. The hairs on the inside of my nostrils are moving and now drenched with her scent. I find the sweet undernote of aroma as my experience unfolds. I become so suffused with this aroma, this lotus essence, that I have become this scent as Kamalāmodamodinī. I am drunk on her.

Lush scent intoxication . . . find some for yourself today. Something floral. Bury your nose in it, bury your whole body in it. Surround yourself in the flowering gifts of Kamalāmodamodinī-Kālī.

47) Kalahaṃsagatiḥ (She Who Is Moving and Swaying with the Gait of a Black Swan)

We are in sacred space, seated with our beloved. We are celebrating union. At some point, in the joyous festivities, it is time to move and dance. Kalahaṃsagatiḥ draws us into the dance, the movement of a swan, and plunges us into certain fulfillment. Having been fully suffused with the blessings of her seat and her scent, intoxicated, we have become Kalahaṃsagatiḥ: the fulfillment. This swan is dancing, black as Kālī (of course), carrying Śiva and Śākti in union sitting together in the lotus, on her back. This process of awakening has such a distinctly feminine feel. This is not a quiet-withdrawn-ascended-overcoming-the-body kind of path. Fully embodied, we feel everything, bring everything to what is unfolding. We dance, we cavort, we sit in sacred circle with others, we feast, we make love, we establish the deities in our bodies: our wild, unruly, delightful, rich, full bodies are the site of it all. Today, as Kalahaṃsagatiḥ, we move and sway supporting union with our bodies. We are the union, and we support the union. We also carry this union back out into the world, in our bodies, as our body. Become it, be it, support it, offer it.

How could anything be separate from this? May it be this way for you as well.

48) Klaibyanāśinī (She Who Is the Destroyer of Fears and Iniquity)

Klaibyanāśinī has arrived just in time, just as everything is all stirred up. Along with this intense delight in our bodies, experienced in the last few names, our darkest hearts, insecurities, vulnerabilities, and fears may be surfacing. We have stirred the pot, the yoni crucible, the cauldron. We are at our edge, if not beyond our edge. Even the soft, sweet, and loving can go too far and become a bit nauseating, I know. The fierce and dark Klaibyanāśinī manifests today to offer us some support. I exhale when a little fierceness is in the room. She will destroy all fears and iniquities if we can offer these to her, place them at her feet. This is her work, far more than your own. It's what she is made for; it is her gift to you. Let her have it all. There is nothing that is too much—too big, or too scary—to ask her to take care of. She's got this, all of it. She knows the depths of our fears and will meet us there, if we only ask her to.

You do not have to struggle alone. Klaibyanāśinī-Kālī is here with you. I'm here. Your spiritual companions are here. You are not alone.

Make offerings. Write down your fears, concerns, insecurities, and all the ways that self-loathing is surfacing as we move into the more subtle realms of this sādhana. Place this piece of paper on your shrine with offerings. In your recitation today, ask Klaibyanāśinī-Kālī to transform them all for you. Ask for her support and love and healing. Let her know that you are in over your head and need to rely on her to see you through. Backing up won't get us through this moment; moving forward, with a heartfelt request to Kālī to take it, will.

This is the moment we have practiced for. In the process of undergoing any sādhana commitment, this moment is guaranteed to arrive if we have given ourselves to the sādhana. This is actually the moment just before the actual transformation begins. We have to bring it all up so that it can be put into the cauldron. Kālī keeps asking: Is there more? Did we leave something out? Lay it all at her feet.

Don't isolate yourselves in the moments of challenge. Connect with loved ones and your spiritual communities. We need each other at moments like this.

49) Kāmarūpiṇī (She Who Is the Form of Desire)

Klaibyanāśinī-Kālī, whom we invoked yesterday, destroys our fears so that we may know what is more true than our fears. What do our fears mask, cover up? Under all the shadow aspects of ourselves, under all the challenges and unhealed aspects, is the simple nature of desire as the pulse of the yoniverse. This is not a nectarine desire, a sweet desire, nor even a socially acceptable desire. This is the nature of desire itself, the intrinsic nature of Kālī's desire, of our desire, of all desire. This is a desire anchored in the nature of the cosmos, the matrix of existence, the web of the yoniverse. This is the desire that will blow us apart and then put us back together. This is the desire that will heal us and give us a place to rest. This is the desire that is her lap. This is the desire for union. This is the union that we merge with at Kāmākhyā, also called Kāmarūpā. The form of desire *is* this body of ours. This body holds and processes, although subtly at times, all polarities. We allow these polarities to be activated by our willingness to engage them, and then we train in how to use them, directing these energies for our spiritual practices. Immersed in the nature of desire, we still live these polarities without identification, thus we can align with either, or both, or neither. We move among all these energies as the flow of all existence.

Polarity, in one form or another, is the spark of desire. Think of how a magnet works. We train in this as a way to connect to the pulse of the yoniverse, so that the microcosm and macrocosm come into union, and then we dissolve like salt in water into the nature of the pulse itself. Pulsing as desire, her desire, desire without reference points; as that which creates/preserves/transforms all in her yoni. This is the pulse of Śakti. Kāmarūpiṇī is the pulse of Śakti. So are we. And the flavor is polarized desire which is, of course, the intrinsic nature of desire. This understanding is at the basis of much of Indic philosophy and all of Tantric experience.

Can you locate the intrinsic nature of desire in your own body, beneath the thoughts, under the fears, beyond all conceptualization? What does it feel like? Is there a temperature, color, movement, emotion? Kāmarūpiṇī flows without any judgments, just the simple presence of the pulse of the intrinsic nature of desire.

50) Kāmarūpakṛtāvāsā (She Who Is Residing at Kāmarūpa, the Very Form of Desire)

A new stanza opens now and we find that we are not just the intrinsic nature of desire, we are residing in the form of desire. The shapeshifting of outer/inner/secret forms continues.

Desire is the movement of the energy of śakti. Śakti is the life-force energy that is the nature of the cosmos, the yoniverse, and desire is the activating energy, the mystery that allows creation to emerge. Desire exists for its own sake. While we may be used to having desire *for*, the form of desire that Kāmarūpakṛtāvāsā shows us is the form of desire for the sake of desire. It just exists. It just is. Cultivating this objectless desire is part of what we do here. And it's no easy task, if my experience is any indication. Some days, it's like wrestling with a huge boa constrictor. Desire just exists as primal energy moving this way and that. Yes, it can be a bit dangerous (watch out for the lashing tail!) and yet this desire just is, the same way that the nature of a boa constrictor just is.

We cultivate desire for its own sake. We take on the form of desire for its own sake. We sit with, we reside with, desire for its own sake. Desire is the fuel for this journey. Our form, her form, is the fuel and vehicle for this journey. When I sit with my huge objectless desire, I want to reach out, to call someone, to *use* the desire for something. Instead, especially when I am on retreat, the sādhana is to sit with the desire and become the form of desire with no object and no activity. Just desire. Sublime. Unexpected. Huge. Ever moving. Just the form of desire.

51) Kāmapīṭhavilāsinī (She Who Is Playing at the Kāmākhyā *Pīṭha*, the Center of the Worship of Desire)

Today, we are all playing at Kāmākhyā's seat, her pīṭha. We are reposing in the center of the worship of desire. This is the form of Kālī that engages in the līlā, the love play, the play of śakti in her home at the Kāmākhyā temple in Assam, India. This is the center, the bindu. At Kāmākhyā, śakti plays more freely than anywhere else. As such, this is also where we worship her as desire. Kāmākhyā is the bindu of our worship of Kālī in her form as desire. Here, as Kāmapīṭhavilāsinī, we join in her cosmic play of desire. Welcome home.

52) Kamanīyā (She Who Is Desired)

Our form is desire, we live as desire, we play with desire, and we are desired. These subtle and multiple shifts of view actually point to the same perception-experience—one that has the potential to draw us into all encompassing love-awareness.

It's one thing to be desire, and desire, and another to have total agency and freedom and be desired. What would it be like to be desired in a way that is not objectifying? What if you knew that being desired wasn't dangerous, but a welcome part of the fabric of existence?

You are desired as the feminine energy in the matrix of union, just as Kamanīyā is. Your being Kamanīyā is a gorgeous gift to the world. You are desired because you bring the gift of feminine energy into existence, and into the world.

Feel into being desired as safe, welcome, available, and healing. Your existence is so sublime that it is desired by all the gods and goddesses. Kamanīyā-Kālī, like you, is so necessary that all existence desires union with her.

Rest in the fullness of being desired.

53) Kalpalatā (She Who Is the Creeper Who Provides Every Desire)

Oh Mā, every desire?

For all of us there will be days when we are so tired, worn out, given, that we just long to take a nap, have some more cookies, and hang with our sakhī for awhile. Yet Mā, with this name, reminds us to continue in latā sādhana, here providing every desire.

Kalpalatā-Kālī knows that we need that rest. But first, she requests one last offering. She invites us to stretch, give, provide, offer from the space of wanting to curl up and hide. *This is the sādhana*—to make the offering even when every fiber of your being says do something else, anything else.

So beloveds, we are here to make the offerings even when we are tender, open, vulnerable, raw, and unbounded: it's like that in latā sādhana sometimes. A practitioner certainly needs a rest. But, there is something more important at stake here, as this name today reveals.

The term *latā* refers to a creeper vine, one of those thick tenacious jungle vines that wraps around a tree, and after some time becomes indivisible from the tree. The term *latā* is also one of the terms for a *female consort* as she is known to wrap herself around her consort the way the creeper wraps around the tree. As the creeper providing every desire (I mean, that's her job description!), we make the offering through our own embodied presencing in latā sādhana. It's truly beautiful. This is the moment we train for. This is what I've given my whole life to be able to do and presence for. This is who I am: Kalpalatā-Kālī. And the offering of every desire to the beloved is what the sādhana is for.

Remember too, beloveds, that this is not the one-sided anonymous offering. This is the mutual matrix-rendition of love and consciousness running through two open bodies as one. I have received as well as offered. I have received far more than I've offered. Just some days, I know that it can be a stretch to keep offering. Maybe it's because I've received so much, that I just want a little time off to integrate it all. Even so, as Mā directs, let me make an offering. My offering to you, dear ones, is the recognition that the creeper is never separate from the tree, the vine never parts from the branch. Only my delusion has me feeling separate. Non-delusion offers non-separateness. Kalpalatā offers this as well.

54) Kamanīyavibhūṣaṇā (She Whose Beauty Is the Ornament)

We have come to the last name of this stanza and now are past the halfway mark in the liturgy. We are fully in the river now, and I can't remember what it was like before we were doing this. In her river, this river of desire life-stream, śakti flowing.

Kamanīyavibhūṣaṇā shows us that our innate natural beauty is a blessing. Our radiant feminine beauty moves out into the world as the presence of grace and love, her grace and her love. Our beauty makes life full, adorned, worth living. Our innate, natural, unencumbered beauty is the manifestation of that which is desired. It might not be overtly desired by everyone, nonetheless it is desire. If we live as this, without waiting for recognition or acknowledgement, as the radiant, beautiful manifestation of all that is desired in the world, we are doing Kamanīyavibhūṣaṇā's work in the world. We bring her into manifestation. As her, the world is full of that which it finds beautiful and that which all desire. This is the source of supreme and divine self-loving, and self-acceptance.

The world tries to tell us differently. Don't believe them. Believe her. Believe Kamanīyavibhūṣaṇā-Kālī.

55) Kamanīyaguṇārādhyā (She Who Is Pleased with the Quality of Tenderness, She Who Is Worshipped with the Quality of Tenderness)

Today our tenderness emerges in response to all that is transpiring. I feel the quality of tenderness that the world offers me in response to my feminine presencing. It is truly a delight to feel the world's tenderness entering me as a gift. Kamanīyaguṇārādhyā also reminds us that not only is our desire and union hot and intense and powerful, it is also tender, subtle, and warming. It nourishes on the cellular level. The whole range of emotions, sensations, and feeling qualities are with us here. After this long run of intense involvement within the center of the lotus, her tenderness is such a relief, and being worshipped with such tenderness is today's gift. Soft, gentle, tender, vulnerable adoration . . . my whole body unfolding into the touch of the beloved. I am grateful to be worshipped tenderly as Kamanīyaguṇārādhyā-Kālī.

This tenderness from others allows me the space for more opening and for integration. Her tenderness is the gift that allows the integration and stabilization of all that has transpired since we began this spiritual practice.

What might Kamanīyaguṇārādhyā's tenderness, and her pleasure at the quality of tenderness around her, offer you today? What healing does it offer, what subtleties? Is there integration that you need? Let it flow through you today as Kamanīyaguṇārādhyā-Kālī's blessing. Feel her tenderness and the tenderness of the world flowing through you, as you. In a world rife with the bold, loud, and large, this is the moment to touch into the tender, quiet, and subtle. Feel yourself as herself there.

56) Komalāṅgī (She Who Is Tender-Bodied)

Our innate tenderness continues today with Komalāṅgī. She is a good reminder that we might be tender today, and so I recommend that you move slowly in the world.

Instead of imagining that Komalāṅgī is about the shape of our physical body, consider this tenderness a description of our subtle body, our inner world. The inner world of winds, channels, and bindu is delicate, and is a tender body-matrix. It is a vast world of immense subtlety, delicacy, and intuitiveness. This is the home of śakti in us. When our inner body is alive and awake, then the channels are open, the winds move, and the bindu circulates. This is the full body love song that I refer to sometimes.

Komalāṅgī is asking us to dive into our own inner experience and trace the lines of awareness in our subtle body. This is not about finding technical diagrams of the energetic body and mapping yours onto it. Please, don't do that. Instead, Komalāṅgī, as the subtle body, is asking us to go inwards and find out what our inner world is like, from our own experience. We go inwards towards our own unerring experience without mapping it onto some formal model. The yoginīs in the Kālīkula know that most of those maps and models were based on some ideal of a male body from the Indic subcontinent. Most of us, even when fully awakened, have a unique and personal form of the subtle body that doesn't match the models. Each of us has a unique, delicate, subtle, tender, inner body matrix. What does yours look like? What is your subtle body like in your womb-yoni-pelvic bowl?

57) Kṛśodarī (She Who Is Slender-Waisted)

How slender is the subtle body? So slender (and of course, tender) that Kṛśodarī is encircling us, no matter the size or shape of our outer form. Kṛśodarī is the waist girdle that brings our awareness into our subtle bodies and anchors it there for our consideration and ongoing reverence. Love this waist as her waist. Love the subtle body that passes between the nose and the perineum, even when you might not have known that it existed before this moment. Love the movement of the waist and belly as we roll the breath through our bodies, tip to toe.

Kṛśodarī-Kālī asks us to feel into the articulation of our waists as the movement of śakti-prāṇā in the body.

Remember the hula hoop? That's Kṛśodarī in big form. Belly rolls are her too. She is the articulation of the upper body with the lower body, the connective stream of bottom to top, top to bottom, side to side. Feel her adorning your midline today. Maybe tie on a waist adornment of some type. Got belly beads? Conch shells on a sacred thread? A slim belt to wear against the skin? A gorgeous scarf? Feel her there as the reminder of the gravitas of your womb that anchors you to the earth and into her love.

58) Kāraṇāmṛtasantoṣā (She Who Is the Cause of the Nectar of Consecrated Wine and Is Also Pleased with It)

A new stanza begins and we flow from the experience of our subtle bodies as divine embodiment into the world of sacred ritual, feasting, and the pañcamakāra. As we've touched on briefly earlier, the pañcamakāra are the five sacred offerings that we make to Kālī and other Tantric deities during pūjā. These pañcamakāra are mentioned in the closing paragraphs of this liturgy (which are not included in the abbreviated version of liturgy that you have here):

> The person who on a new moon night, when it falls on a Tuesday, worships the great Ādyā Kālī, Mistress of the Three Worlds, with the five makāras [37]// and repeats her hundred names, becomes suffused with the presence of Kālī, and for this person there remains nothing in the Three Worlds which is beyond their powers. [38]//

These five makāras include consecrated wine which is offered to Kālī.

This consecrated wine offering to Kālī Mā is the body offering of Kāraṇāmṛtasantoṣā. This consecrated wine is understood as analogous to nectar—it is the nectar that emerges in our bodies as a result of our dedication to Kālī, our practice, our offering; the nectar that flows through the nether mouth as desire arises. Kāraṇāmṛtasantoṣā is the inner love-bliss-freedom-awareness that causes the nectar to arise and flow. The consecrated wine is not separate from this. The nectar brings a kind of bliss-intoxication that allows a little softer union to be present. The nectar flows as a result of union. It's all bliss-freedom in this cup. Kāraṇāmṛtasantoṣā brings forth this nectar and is pleased with it. Can you imagine, for a moment, in conventional reality, how pleasing yoni-nectar might be?

Run with this. Practice with this. Find the nectars that please Kāraṇāmṛtasantoṣā-Kālī and make them an offering on your shrine to her.

59) Kāraṇānandasiddhidā (She Who Gives *Siddhi* to Those Who Rejoice in Consecrated Wine)

We are fully in the realm of Kāraṇānandasiddhidā with the offerings of consecrated wine at our shrines. When we find ourselves here, and partake of the wine as her, we find that we are rejoicing. Here is the pleasure. Here is the softening. Here is the union.

In this union with her, we discover that we are not who we thought we were. There is a sense that we are more than our ordinary selves at play. Our extraordinary selves have emerged, and we are taking our seats. Here, in the realm of the extraordinary, when we know we are more than our small selves, we find that the normal rules of life don't apply. We find that we are more than we ever knew. In this state, with this knowing, we have entered into the world of *siddhi** where extraordinary things are always possible. This is the blessing of Kāraṇānandasiddhidā-Kālī: knowing that extraordinary things are within the realm of possibility. As you rejoice today, know that this is the siddhi, the blessing that she offers us in return for our devotion and commitment. Let her cups of nectar take you where you need to go.

60) Kāraṇānandajāpeṣṭā (She Who Is the Deity of Those Who Do *Japa* When Joyed with Consecrated Wine)

Today's name reminds us that we are in the womb-heart of her worship now. We are in deep, in the middle of this sādhana. It's like being in the middle of the middle of the middle. Kāraṇānandajāpeṣṭā emerges in the middle portion of any single offering of a Tantric sādhana or pūjā. Here she is emerging not just to let us know we are in the middle of a single offering of her sādhana, but to remind us we are also in just that far in our 108 recitations of Kālī's 100 names. The middle of the middle of the middle. We are in it so deeply that when I look over at the Kālī shrine, I can't remember a time when we weren't doing this together. It's like some huge flashback/flash forward/all time thing—right here in her yoni crucible, with all of you, offering her sādhana together.

In a full Tantric sādhana, after the offerings, prayers, the saṅkalpa, and the *dhyāna** (meditation visualization), there is japa and the offering of the pañcamakāra (five sacred feast offerings). Perhaps you made the offerings of the pañcamakāra at your Kālī shrine on the first night of this sādhana together. As I noted a few entries ago, it's part of the undertaking of this *Song of the Hundred Names of Ādyā Kālī*.

So, here we are, at the point in the practice when we have offered Kālī the pañcamakāra and have ourselves partaken in the feast. We are joyed now. The bliss and freedom run strongly here. We are with our beloved (in whatever form that is today), and we are in love. We are her love. We are her. We are reciting her mantra with love and awareness moving freely in us. We are relaxed, happy, in union with all of it.

We begin the recitation of her mantra to bring her even closer, and now know we are Kāraṇānandajāpeṣṭā inseparably. I can't imagine being anywhere else but right here, with all of you . . . for as long as we are, for as long as it takes, no one left behind.

61) Kāraṇārcanaharṣitā (She Who Is Glad to Be Worshipped with Consecrated Wine)

How could we not be glad to be worshipped with consecrated wine? It sounds ideal to me; what else is there? Well, maybe garlands made out of jasmine flowers. Otherwise, this is so full and complete. We set out the items for worship, we worship our beloved as the deity, we become the deity, and we are also worshipped with the consecrated wine. This gladdens me immeasurably, here in the middle of the middle of the middle. All the nuances of how we presence during sādhana are here. We make offerings, we worship, we remember our inseparability with deity, and then we are worshipped because we are her, as Kāraṇārcanaharṣitā. This makes me so happy that I'm overflowing. This is the moment we've been waiting for. This is the moment of completion, union, fulfillment, right here in the middle of the middle of the middle.

I am not only gladdened by this worship, I am grateful for it. My entire DNA structure changed as I absorbed the worship of others; when I was worshipped as Kālī, everything changed. My body rewired to take in this truth. Can you drink in this truth? Can you embody Kāraṇārcanaharṣitā and let the consecrated wine move through you so fully that your molecular structure, the fiber of your being, the matrix of your yoniverse changes? Fall open into this love with me.

62) Kāraṇārṇavasammagnā (She Who Is Immersed in an Ocean of Consecrated Wine)

The blessings continue. I'm almost drowning in the splendor of this ocean of her love. "Consecrated wine" is actually just part of that Tantric twilight language (sandhyā bhāṣā), and also refers to both her amṛta and her intoxicating love for us. This wine, which we initially blessed at the beginning of the sādhana, is now being offering to us. In it is her love and commitment to us. We drink this consecrated wine until we are suffused in Kāraṇārṇavasammagnā's love. We are fully immersed in her ocean of love. We are her love. We are her. We are so fully immersed, here in this middle place, that it suffuses every cell of our bodies. Every pore is full of her love wine. We are drinking it in through our skin. We are gulping it down as nourishment until there is no part of us that is untouched by her. Her amṛta-wine flows into us from every place, and we take it in from every place. Immersed. Drenched. Suffused. Take it in fully. The moment is now.

63) Kāraṇavratapālinī (She Who Protects Those Who Accomplish *Vrata* with Consecrated Wine)

Yesterday, we were suffused, immersed in her ocean of love. According to the *Kulārṇava Tantra*, we have earned the right to call ourselves *yoginī* and/or *yogi*.

Because she practices the yoni-mudrā,
attends upon the Feet of Girija (the Divine Mother),
and because of the glory of total immergence[3] without support,
she is called yoginī.
O My Beloved!
Because he throbs with the glory of the Mantra due to the practice of yoni-mudrā
and because he is adorable to the host of deities,
he is called yogi.

This feels so alive and vibrant today. This is where we are, immersed and immerged.

Now we go further. Here, we see the benefit of dedicating ourselves to her practices. Here, with Kāraṇavratapālinī, we come back to this again: because we will eventually *accomplish* her practices, she protects us. Let me explain.

A *vrata** is a commitment to spiritual practice (like the sādhana of reciting her names). It is undertaken to achieve blessings of one's desires, as well as to mature in spiritual awareness. It can potentially move us more dynamically into union with full embodied awakening. Technically, *vrata* means *to vow* or *promise*. The term *vrata* also sometimes carries the taste of making a sacrifice or promise to the goddess in order to achieve one's aims.

Here, at name sixty-three, we discover that we are accomplishing our vrata together (no one left behind) with her consecrated wine-nectar, and thus, Kāraṇavratapālinī is our protectress. She is with us inseparably as our guardian; ever near, ever watchful, ever protective. We can rest in this with great comfort. Can you feel her protective energies filling you, surrounding you? It is part of the ocean of her amṛta-love that we have been immersed in. They go together.

64) Kastūrīsaurabhāmodā (She Who Is Gladdened by the Scent of Musk)

Her sixty-fourth name! This is a stunningly gorgeous and auspicious number to go with a glorious and auspicious name. In these sacred goddess traditions, the number sixty-four is associated with the divine feminine and her manifestations. The sixty-fourth name brings us to a moment of celebration and alignment.

After we offer, and imbibe, and immerse in the offering of consecrated amṛta-wine ever so fully, in the ripeness of our pūjā, we move into union. Now, we meet our beloved, our desire rises and musk flows as union intensifies. The scent fills the shrine room. Kastūrīsaurabhāmodā is gladdened. We are making the offering. In fact, we are the offering.

65) Kastūrītilakojjvalā (She Who Is the Luminous One with a *Tīlaka* of Musk)

The musk is flowing in our sādhana-pūjā with our beloved. Union is intense, wild, real. We are warm, energies are moving intensely. A warm flush is all around and we are glowing a little, almost perspiring. We are happy, in her lap. We collect a little of that musk on our ring finger and apply the *tilaka** as adornment and blessing to our third eye and to the third eye of the beloved. The air pressure in the room shifts and everything glows and twinkles with the light display of love-bliss-awareness-consciousness-Kālī. We feel, as Kastūrītilakojjvalā, how there is a far greater reality, love-matrix-field, beyond the conventional reality that we are normally inhabiting. We have crossed over, and we are joyous and luminous. We feel and understand now. We have a taste of what this might all be about.

66) Kastūrīpūjanaratā (She Who Rejoices in the Worship with Musk)

Now that I have musk dripping down the middle of my forehead . . . .

Kastūrīpūjanaratā loves this part. Drippy, messy, wet, luminous, warm union with the beloved, surrounded by the pañcamakāra. Jasmine garlands in our hair, musk being offered in worship, while we drop into union again and again. Our senses are fully alive now. We are relaxed. We are full of bliss-awareness and passing it back and forth with our beloved. Moving love and freedom into the room through open bodies. Kastūrīpūjanaratā rejoices.

Perhaps you can find a little musk today and find a way to offer it in worship of her? What might this look like? What might this feel like?

67) Kastūrīpūjakapriyā (She Who Loves Those Who Worship Her with Musk)

Can you feel her love?

We are in full worship of her, with musk dripping off our foreheads. Amṛta is all around us. We have opened enough, offered enough, dropped in enough, found enough union to be able to finally feel her wild unconditional love for us. Can you feel the love-matrix of the yoniverse pulsing all around, through you, as you? Can you feel the yoniverse, Kālī, Kastūrīpūjakapriyā loving you? Can you receive this love into your body? Take another inhalation and let her love-śakti permeate your being. Let her love drench you. Receive this love blessing into every nook, cranny, corner, shadow, depth, flowing part of yourself. Drink this in. She loves you. Always. Unconditionally.

68) Kastūrīdāhajananī (She Who Is Mother of Those Who Burn Musk as Incense)

Mā just keeps loving us. Can you feel her love? This love is so grand, so unremitting, so wild, free, and unstoppable, that we know her as our mother. Kālī is our mother, the mother we never had. Kastūrīdāhajananī takes us in her arms and offers us the love we miss, the love we pushed away, the love we never had, the love we crave, the love we are. She is the mother of the universe, all existence. She is that vast. She is also exceedingly personal, intimate, our own mother. Kastūrīdāhajananī-Kālī is the poignancy of re-mothering for us in every moment.

We are in the midst of a shift from sexual desire and union with the beloved, to mother and mothering. A new face, a new flow, in union with the beloved, whatever is unattended to arises just as in the deepest lovemaking and the deepest intimacy. This is the deepest lovemaking and the deepest intimacy. Kālī is holding us in this, in all these roles and ways. In union, our heart-womb-pelvis arises and makes known what is unhealed, what is not whole, what we need. Right now, we are being held in her arms, being offered all we need. The flavor is Kastūrīdāhajananī. The flavor is mother. This is sublime.

Perhaps you can burn some musk incense at your shrine today, right now, as an offering to her?

69) Kastūrīmṛgatoṣiṇī (She Who Is Fond of the Musk Deer)

She is exceedingly happy with anything that offers musk, creates musk, exudes musk. We have been making full-bodied offerings of musk to Kālī in many forms over these last days. Kastūrīmṛgatoṣiṇī reminds us that it's not just our musk that she is fond of, but all the forms and sources of musk that can be found. She actually makes no distinction. Our musk, their musk, musk from a musk deer, musk from an elephant in rut, the rich unforgettable smell of animals in heat, and of us when we are heated up. She is fond of it all.

Musk, from musk deer, is also the base of many of the most sensual perfumes, and is one of the most expensive animal products on the planet. The gland that exudes this musk is only found in adult males, and lies between their genitals and belly button. So perfect that it comes from this same pelvic region that we treasure, and the focus of so much of our spiritual practice here.

So rarified is authentic musk that it is worth a queen's ransom. Imagine, the rich depth and intensity of our musk is that valuable. In this world, it is. It's the amṛta-nectar-ichor that lets us know we are moving into the realms where the most secret Tantric transformations are possible.

In addition, based on wisdom in other lineages, musk from the musk deer is understood as a powerful medicine that brings important healing in the Tantric worldview. This healing allows us to actually undertake and establish the foundations of a Tantric spiritual life.

Kastūrīmṛgatoṣiṇī-Kālī is so fond of the musk deer, who offers us this musk for our own healing, sensual adornment, and union offerings. In her honor, perhaps you can spread a little musk around your space, put some on your body, generate some musk and make it an offering. This is full-bodied Tantric practice.

70) Kastūrībhojanaprītā (She Who Is Pleased to Eat the Musk of the Musk Deer)

Reading this name, I can do nothing but laugh out loud, and I feel such great delight at her wisdom. This is the form of Kālī who is pleased to eat the musk of the musk deer. We might imagine that Kastūrībhojanaprītā is doing this for health reasons, given that the musk from the musk deer has healing properties. Yet, in my mind, full of Tantric twilight language, and double and triple entendre, I have gone far further than that. I hope you do too. Kastūrībhojanaprītā is our beloved and our musk is flowing.

71) Karpūrāmodamoditā (She Who Is Gladdened by the Scent of Camphor)

From musk to camphor, from offering incense to offering camphor. We make all these esoteric offerings as a token of our love and gratitude to Kālī in all her forms. Just as we offer to a Kumārī what will please her, so too we offer to Kālī what pleases her. Kālī is the form of Karpūrāmodamoditā when she is gladdened by the scent of camphor being offered in the room.

Camphor is one of the precious offerings used in worship. It comes in small blocks, and we place a tiny piece on a special ritual implement accompanied by the ringing of a bell. We light it and offer this pure clear flame to Kālī. Camphor is renowned for burning with no residue; it is an offering of light and blessings that is clean and clear. The burning of camphor allows us to offer a clear divine flame to Kālī and to bless ourselves as well. Camphor is also thought to be cooling, which for a hot goddess like Kālī is important.

Perhaps there is something in your life that could use a little cooling right now? Is there some unresolved anger, a fever, some blistering "something" that might be eased through the offering of cooling camphor? Making this offering to our own heat as her heat pleases Karpūrāmodamoditā-Kālī to no end. I'll offer camphor flame at my shrine tonight.

72) Karpūramālābharaṇā (She Who Is Adorned with Garlands of Camphor)

Karpūramālābharaṇā is sitting with us here in pūjā. Right here, knee to knee, eye to eye, offering rose petals to each other with each name, each mantra, each bite of the pañcamakāra, each sip is sublime suffusion of immergence into her love. Things have gotten so hot for me here, so heated, that instead of just offering the flame of camphor, I have strung together a gorgeous garland of chunks of camphor for her to wear around her neck to cool her down a little. Here, Mā, let me offer you this . . . on behalf of all who participate in this ritual.

We want to *burn*, yes, just not *burn up* before we have given everything we have incarnated to give. We want to burn steadily, incandescently, sublimely, on fire with her love. Sometimes we have to tend the fire to cool it off a little bit so that we are in for the long slow burn. I haven't finished the offerings of this lifetime, Karpūramālābharaṇā-Kālī, and a little cooling right now will help me keep going without combusting. Mā, please take this garland of camphor so we can keep going.

Has something gotten too hot (or too cold?) for you to keep going? If so, perhaps you might offer a little camphor today to Karpūramālābharaṇā-Kālī in support of a little cooling off (or warming up) to all of this, to her, to her names, to this sādhana, to your practice, to your devotion to her, to your offering.

Mā, please, take my offerings. I am at your feet burning up with desire for union without end.

73) Karpūracandanokṣitā (She Whose Body Is Smeared with Camphor and Sandalpaste)

This next wondrous name, with all that it implies, naturally emerges from the ritual of union we experienced with the previous one. I write this commentary on the morning after, and the plates haven't been cleared yet. The shrine is overflowing with the offerings. Incense has burnt all the way down and the wine cups are drained down to the dregs. There is sindur caked on my third eye, kohl smeared down my cheeks, and my sari is twisted and rumpled. What is that stuck on the back of my sari? My beloved, Karpūracandanokṣitā, is covered with the offerings of camphor and sandalpaste that I made last night with my own hands. I have indeed lovingly smeared my beloved's body with all that is here. I couldn't keep my hands off her, I couldn't keep to the script. No wonder I have matted hair and that distinctive morning-after taste in my mouth. I am sure I did not floss or neti before I fell asleep in her lap last night.

I'm bleary this morning, and being gentle with myself as is necessary when we emerge from such union. Going so slowly as the dawn breaks. The pink and orange sky feels like a gentle reminder of the blessings of this practice. I stand outside under the morning sky holding my beloved's hand, ever united in the perfume of sandalwood and camphor. We don't say a word.

74) Karpūrakāraṇāhlādā (She Who Is Pleased with Consecrated Wine with Camphor)

Karpūrakāraṇāhlādā's consecrated wine is so fine. The consecrated wine with camphor that we have shared during our pūjā of union has my head reeling. So sublime are the utter subtleties of this pūjā. Nothing is straightforward, and nothing left out.

Take a moment today to sense how far we have come in our sādhana together. We are almost three-fourths of the way through. As we begin to transition into the final nights, the last three weeks of our time together, I'd invite you to feel your own pleasure in this sādhana. Find some piece of this practice that gives you pleasure. When you find that pleasure, linger there and intensify your pleasure. As we move through these final nights, move through the names with lingering pleasure. This is the sensual feast of union with our beloved. Let yourself find pleasure and satisfaction in these last days as we take in the last drops of depth sādhana, notice the softness in everyone's gaze, and feel the freedom, love and bliss moving through us. Drink in this moment. The consecrated wine with camphor that is Karpūrakāraṇāhlādā's amṛta is sublime and pulsing in my mouth.

75) Karpūrāmṛtapāyinī (She Who Drinks the Nectar with Camphor)

Who is drinking what with whom? Karpūrāmṛtapāyinī lifts her cup to sip the last of the wine we offered during the pūjā. She is still wearing her garland of camphor. I am still wearing my jasmine flower garland. I feel how the union persists even as I move around the room softly adjusting to the daylight. She drinks, and passes the last sip to me. I drink in this last sip of amṛta and can taste her camphor on the cup.

What form of Kālī is this who sips nectar with camphor with me? What form of Kālī are you? What form of Kālī is all manifest existence?

76) Karpūrasāgarasnātā (She Who Is Bathed in the Ocean of Camphor)

I drink in the last of the nectar with camphor with my beloved Karpūrasāgarasnātā. It is so powerful, so dynamic, that I begin to be suffused in it. The nectar moves through me and penetrates all of me. I fall into Karpūrasāgarasnātā-Kālī's amṛta. I am drunk again, and am swimming in it internally; no part of me is untouched by the sublime movement of this nectar. I look around and find that the internal nectar has become the external nectar. The air and energies around us are bathed in this. We are bathing in her ocean of camphor. We are so suffused in such union that all of existence is her nectar-amṛta infused with the heady camphor. I surrender to this experience knowing that there is nowhere else I'd rather be. Instead of fighting, I allow myself to just float. I don't disappear into unconsciousness; I float and am aware of being in the ocean of camphor and watching the ocean of camphor. Karpūrasāgarasnātā begins to wash her body, bathing without a trace of self-consciousness.

77) Karpūrasāgarālayā (She Who Is at Home in the Ocean of Camphor)

She is so at home here in this ocean, so at peace. We float together, surrendered to this ocean of camphor. I know that here I can rest. I am at home. She is at home. This is her element, her ocean, her way. Another way to describe this "place" might be to say that it is also her lap. Her lap holds this ocean of camphor-nectar-union-surrender-bliss-freedom that I can't live without. So I adjust my internal and external worlds, drop my preferences and preconceptions and expectations. I just let myself float here with Karpūrasāgarālayā. We are stretched out on these waters, near to each other. I can feel her breathing me through the ocean.

78) Kūrcabījajapaprītā (She Who Is Pleased When Worshipped with the Recitation of the Bīja *Hūṁ*)

A new stanza and a new run of names. This stanza moves us into another realm entirely, a quick transit from the end of the pūjā and dissolving into the ocean, to more specifics about worship of Kālī. Flowing, floating into this next arising.

Kūrcabījajapaprītā is the form of Kālī who loves to be worshipped with the bīja mantra *hūṁ*. While Kālī's most common bīja is *krīṃ*, other bīja make their way into our worship and practice, depending on what is needed in the moment. The relevance of *hūṁ* will make itself known soon enough. For now, know that Kūrcabījajapaprītā is pleased to have *hūṁ* recited in our worship of her. And when the goddess is pleased, how can we not also feel her pleasure as our own? All is right in the yoniverse at moments like this when we are resting in the simple grace of her pleasure.

Can you move into the grace of your own pleasure today? What is your experience? Can you find a bodily experience of pleasure and a way to link it to her pleasure?

79) Kūrcajāpaparāyaṇā (She Who Threatens and Conquers Demons by Muttering *Hūṁ*)

Our shadow and wounding are with us on this journey. No one left behind, nothing left behind. It's all included. All of it. All of us. When our wounding, our shadow, our projections begin to get in the way, overwhelm us, threaten to have us flailing in the ocean of her nectar, it's time to bring out the mantras for support and to cut through. Part of Kālī's nature is to carry a sword of truth that cuts away all that keeps us separate. This sword of truth helps us to regain our equanimity in the midst of the battlefield of our own psyche and our life. Reciting one of her powerful mantras, *hūṁ*, can offer us the steadiness and stability of Kūrcajāpaparāyaṇā. The mantra is her form. It is her.

Recite it quickly and feel the sound of bees buzzing through your body as this unfolds. Feel her vibration moving through you and bringing you back to union with yourself and with her. Let *hūṁ* cut through all forms of separation. Remember yourself as her form.

80) Kulīnā (She Who Is the Embodiment of the Kulācāra, the Kula Teachings)

The eightieth name . . . We are in the final portion of our sādhana. Please, keep going. It might be difficult, unwanted, or even boring by now, but please keep going. For the sake of the whole kula of yoginīs and yogis who have committed to this recitation of the *Song of the Hundred Names of Ādyā Kālī*, please keep going.

Today's name, Kulīnā, is the embodiment of the *kulācārā*,* the kula teachings, the teachings of the Kālīkula. Kulīnā says here at the eightieth name, on the eightieth name, that our perseverance and dedication and devotion have fashioned us into the nature of the kula teachings. The teachings are inseparable from the kula itself, just as Kālī is inseparable from her names. We are the embodiment of the kula. How could we not be? The kula is the Tantric clan of family who share in devotion to Kālī. We are the embodiments of the left-handed path, however it manifests today, right here where we live, as we live. There are no strict rules of membership, there are no guidelines, nor codes of conduct. We are here, in the Kālīkula because we love Kālī and have dedicated ourselves to her practice. This is Kulīnā-Kālī: dedicated, in love, embodied, devoted, blazing in union whenever possible.

81) Kaulikārādhyā (She Who Is Adored by the Kaulika, the Practitioners of Kulācāra)

She is the embodiment of the kulācāra, she is the kulācāra. We love her as inseparable from the teachings and practice and community. Can you "read" her body, her form, as the sādhana liturgy? Can you read her every name as practice instruction? Her form is the teachings. Kaulikārādhyā's form is the sādhana. Her form is the gurvī. Her breath is our heartbeat. We adore her for this. We adore her as this. All form is thus, and we adore her thus.

82) Kaulikapriyakāriṇī (She Who Is the Benefactress of the Practitioners of the Kaulika, the Cause of the Love [of the Kaulika for the Kulācāra])

Our love of the kula and of Ādyā Kālī in all her forms allows us to come into relationship with her in a loving give-and-take relationship. Here, we discover that we are well cared for. Not just loved, but well cared for. Kaulikapriyakāriṇī is our protector and benefactress. She cares for our well being on so many levels that we can't even name them all.

I'm sure that Kaulikapriyakāriṇī is taking care of me. I have a warm place to live, enough food, and soft sheets. That's her blessing and protection. I am well loved, and have the chance to love like crazy. Oh Kaulikapriyakāriṇī Mā, thank you. Your support of my life is a great benefit, and I am so grateful, so crazy grateful. This is all hers, and look at how rich and full my life is with her! Oh Mā, I get it. Your blessings, grace, and care infuse everything I do. I might need to put out more offerings, and practice more. I might need to love harder and wilder. I might need to be just a touch happier. All because she brings so much to my life! Can you look at your life and carefully note five ways that she is caring for you? Ten things? Make a crazy list of 108 things and see what emerges.

83) Kulācārā (She Who Is Observant of the Kulācāra)

Kulācārā observes the ways of the kulācāra. Again, we see that she is the form of herself. Every name is her form. Every form is her name. She is not separate from her name. Nor are we. She is herself, utterly.

She is a Tantrika. She practices the ways of the Kālīkula. She observes the ways of the left-handed Tantric practitioners. Our way towards her is to follow the path she offers. And so we undertook the *Song of the Hundred Names of Ādyā Kālī*. All differences disappear, folding in onto themselves. This is union upon union.

84) Kautukinī (She Who Is the Joyous One)

How can we be joyous in the midst of suffering? The challenges of life and love and embodiment are enough to have most of us thinking that simple happiness and joy are not possible for us, not now, not under these conditions. Kautukinī tells us otherwise. We don't become happy because the external conditions change; we become happy, joyous even, when we decide that is how we want to go through life. This isn't a false happiness, nor a gliding over of the challenges. It is a state of internal knowing that, even in the midst of all the awful, Kautukinī-Kālī is with us. We are not separate from our beloved. Never. Not ever. Can you feel under all the conditioning, preconceptions, habits, experiences, and find a thread of connection to her, to your beloved? Focus on that thread of her lovelight as though it were your lifeline; it is the trail of bread crumbs, the hand in the dark. Focus on the thread of connection, and let it grow. We have been undertaking this liturgy with just this purpose. Let it grow. Remember this connection, remember her. She is joyous with us, in us, as us. Her joy is ours.

85) Kulamārgapradarśinī (She Who Is the Revealer of the Kula Path to Seekers)

She reveals the path . . . . Can you sense this? Feel her as the path? You seek and she has responded, opening up and offering you the nature of your heart's desire. Rest now. She is the path we seek.

86) Kāśīśvarī (She Who Is the Supreme Goddess of Kāśī-Varanasi)

Varanasi (aka Benares aka Kāśī) is one of the most sacred cities on the planet. Varanasi is to many Hindus what Rome is to many Catholics. The most sacred river, the Ganges (or Gaṅgā) runs here, and her banks are dotted with *ghāṭs,** the places where human cremations take place. Kālī is highly revered here as the supreme goddess. Kāśī is a dirty city, a wild chaotic swirl of all existence. The Gaṅgā is one of the most polluted rivers on the planet, and yet demonstrates the miracle of pink dolphins jumping in her waves at dusk. Kāśī-Varanasi is rough and tumble and sublime, full of death and celebration. Her kind of place for sure. Ganges is her river (and thus she is one with Gaṅgā Mā), and her pollution, and her trash, and her Śiva, and her whirlwind of life and death, all mixed up together. Truly this is one of her sacred seats.

87) Kaṣṭahartrī (She Who Removes Difficulties, Sufferings)

This sādhana has not necessarily been easy for us. So many difficulties, arisings, challenges. Life can be hard. Yet we have the freedom and blessings to practice. As female practitioners, as female devotees, as female lovers, we have more freedom and opportunity to practice than almost any other women on the planet. We are fortunate. As are the men of the Kālīkula. The freedom and willingness to practice offers us opportunities to handle the challenges in our lives with more openness, willingness, acceptance, and ease. Kaṣṭahartrī does not take away the actual difficulties (at least not always), yet she does offer us the opportunity to drop into her graceful mind where we can handle all the challenges with more of the qualities that make them easier to weather. We aren't disengaging here; we are fully engaging with clarity, perspective, love, and acceptance. Kaṣṭahartrī allows us to be present and full of love with whatever is happening. In this, we know ourselves as her, with her. She is in us, supporting us towards love and clarity in our lives. Union with her makes the ongoing challenges of life far less difficult.

Ask Kaṣṭahartrī-Kālī to take away your difficulties today. Offer all your challenges into her lap. Give away your attachment to holding the challenges in the particular way that you are holding them. Ask her to offer new perspectives on what is transpiring. Ask her to help you hold it all with love and presence . . . and a little lightness too.

88) Kāśīśavaradāyinī (She Who Is the Giver of Blessings to Śiva, Lord of Kāśī-Varanasi)

Yes, she blesses Lord Śiva. God receives blessings from goddess. This name indicates the Śākta Tantric worldview at play. In other forms of Tantra, and in mainstream Hinduism, normally Śiva or the other gods bless everyone and everything, including goddesses. Not so here. This name draws together the primordial qualities of Ādyā Kālī and brings them into play in the place, Kāśī-Varanasi, where, within other worldviews, Śiva is the ultimate deity. He might be the lord of Kāśī, yet that is not enough. Not in this liturgy nor in the Kālīkula. I embrace Śiva, but it's Śakti who is the ultimate form of ultimate truth; she is primordial here, not he. As such, as the womb-matrix of all reality, she offers the blessings of existence to the others. She is the blessing force of the primordial womb. This is her. This is us.

89) Kāśīśvarakṛtāmodā (She Who Is the Giver of Pleasure to the Lord of Kāśī)

pleasure	reciting
desire	receiving
offering	dropping
blessing	holding

pushing	biting
pulling	kissing
opening	licking
closing	delivering
opening	pulling back
scratching	pleasure

This is union upon union on this blessed day. It is a perfect day to do a longer and slower recitation of her names, savoring the sensual and erotic pleasures of her hundred forms. Perhaps you might even do some extra recitations to offer to others, and to receive extra blessings for yourself and your family.

90) Kāśīśvaramanorama (She Who Is the Beloved of the Lord of Kāśī, She Who Overwhelms His Mind with Beauty)

Our minds . . . sigh. It sure is noisy some days. My mind and intellect have been such gifts in my life and on this journey. And, there are times when my focus of leading from the mind has constricted and masculinized me. When I was in graduate school I was rigid, and thought I could think my way through all of life; I thought I could control it all to avoid my own suffering. My mind and the confusion of my thoughts was just so loud: the thoughts, the judgments, the self-critique, the self-loathing. So little of it was relevant or true. Maybe none of it was. Yet my mind was so ridiculously noisy, taking in so much information that I was allowing to take me in quite the wrong directions. Meditation and sādhana were a joy to me because they helped to quiet my mind, and helped to loosen the hold of the negative thought patterns. What a gift this has been to quiet the doubts and self-loathing through the recitation of her mantras and her names.

Over time, my mind got quieter and something else happened. I began to feel into how Kālī was slowly and ceaselessly showing me a new way of being. She was showing me a new way of thinking about myself. She showed me a way of knowing who I truly was/am underneath the life-long habit of negative thoughts. She overwhelmed my mind with the beauty of the divine feminine. She overwhelmed me with beauty. She showed me that every woman was her and every woman was beautiful and loved. I was too. I was not left out of that generalization. She showed me over and over how to allow my negative self-image to be replaced by an authentic, positive self-regard and self-love. Not a surface assertion of "I'm beautiful" or "I'm a goddess," but a wild, unfettered understanding of my true nature. Every bit of me is loved and every bit of me is her. Remembering this as I watch my body age, when I see unflattering photos, when I say or do ungraceful or outright ugly things, this is her overwhelming my mind with love, truth, bliss, and freedom. Her splendor, her grace, her love is so much more powerful than my negative thought patterns. Her splendor heals this. She has overwhelmed my mind and I wouldn't have it any other way.

91) Kalamañjīracaraṇā (She Whose Toe Bells Make Sweet Melodies as She Moves)

Our minds are soft and clear, and now we can begin to move into the world as love and beauty. The gift of the feminine is to manifest love as beauty in the world.

Adornment is not just for our own body sādhana (as we have been discussing), but also for the movement of beauty into the world. We offer beauty through our bodies, as our bodies, as our spirit, our heart-wombs, our ways: all of our ways, no matter the flavor. Our adornment is an embodied reminder of the beauty we are, and that we are that beauty as we move. Let yourself find a way into your body today, perhaps a way that you haven't before, so that your whole being wafts sweet melodies of love and beauty as you move. Let this be the offering.

92) Kvaṇatkāñcīvibhūṣaṇā (She Whose Girdle Bells Sweetly Tinkle)

Her hips sway and the girdle bells tinkle, moving more feminine grace and beauty out into the world. Kvaṇatkāñcīvibhūṣaṇā has a powerfully activated pelvis and she moves it with intention and elegance so that the śakti swirls and the girdle bells do their magic.

What would it be like to wear girdle bells? Can you imagine what kind of awareness would be drawn to your pelvis if you did this? Can you imagine how present and seductive you might feel, in your own body? All the best statues of yoginīs that I've seen include impressive waist belts holding the energy of the hips down, pressing the weight into the feet and connecting her with the earth. Can you imagine moving in the world like this? What's all this śakti flowing so close to the end of the sādhana? What purpose might this serve? What offering is this? What sādhana is being revealed?

93) Kāñcanādrikṛtāgārā (She Who Is Residing in the Golden Mountain, Mount Meru)

A week until we are complete with her names. Ten nights until we finish the sādhana. Please remember that while the contemplation of her names will finish with the hundredth name, you may have committed to 108 recitations of the *Song of the Hundred Names of Ādyā Kālī*. Feel into what it means to be coming into completion with this sādhana. Feel into the fullness of where we have been, and the fullness of these final days. What has changed for you? What has transformed?

She is well-adorned feminine love and beauty moving out into the world. She is also fully seated at Mount Meru, the center of the universe. She is in all aspects of worldly life, and she is seated in the center of her yantra. Mount Meru is not just a place, it is also the central yantra that comprises all manifest and unmanifest existence. She is there, in the center of that. Kañcanādrikṛtāgārā is in the bindu of this yantra. She is the bindu of this yantra. She lives in this yantra as the yantra. Her seat is the cosmic bindu from which all existence issues forth, and into which it comes back. This is the os of the cervix. She resides there. Can you sense her residing in the os of your cervix? What is your bodily experience when you feel into that? What if you moved from there? Can you see where the waist girdle is leading us? What would it be like to move from our energetic center, the bindu-os where Kālī lives? Perhaps you would like to try doing this today and tonight? I live from there as much as possible . . . it changes everything.

94) Kāñcanācalakaumudī (She Who Is the Shining Moonbeam on the Mountain of Gold, She Who Displays Radiant Wealth on Her Top Cloth)

We have come to the last name in this stanza; we have come to the end of the end now. She is Meru, she resides in Meru, her seat is the yantra-Meru, and she is the glistening light of the moon shining down onto Meru. The boat-of-heaven crescent moon was up the night before I wrote this contemplation, and the bright light of her blessings glimmered down as I walked the cold streets. Kāñcanācalakaumudī's light is the wealth—the true wealth of creation—a sparkling, reflective, lunar light dance.

There was a time before existence, then all coalesced into energy-bindu. As she gave birth to it (remember that gorgeous squatting goddess?), the first tendrils of existence that emerged were as light. Just light. Gorgeous sparkling lunar light. This is the radiant wealth that she wears on top of her sari. It is not just an inner light, but an offering of that light visibly outwards.

Perhaps Kāñcanācalakaumudī-Kālī is suggesting that we wear our hearts on our sleeves today.

95) Kāmabījajapānandā (She Who Is in Complete Bliss to Hear the Recitation of the Bīja Mantra *Klīṃ*)

This is the last stanza; we are moving into the final moments of the perfection of the sādhana. As I write this, I am moved by the melancholy in my system: our sādhana is coming to an end. Perhaps it's a night to recite *klīṃ* then . . . to gladden Kāmabījajapānandā-Kālī-Kāmākhyā and myself too. This takes us into the seed-heart-womb-bīja of it all. *Ānanda* also means absolute bliss, complete joy, or delight. I am in complete and absolute joy and bliss because I recite her bīja mantra. Ahhhhhhhhhhhh that feels so luscious and alive. Melancholy and bliss moving together; this is truly her way.

Klīṃ.

❁ ❁ ❁

This sādhana of the recitation of the *Song of the Hundred Names of Ādyā Kālī* is powerful, and like all Kālī sādhanas, it will bring to the surface that which is unhealed and needs tending.

What I have noticed in leading groups through this practice is that there is a larger process that unfolds. Our shadow may rise up, and we may be stepping into healing of old unhealed wounds. We may be sick in various ways, or feeling "triggered" and even "re-traumatized." Given that we are near the end of our sādhana, and it has been a long collective journey, I will not be surprised. It is typical for things to intensify near the end of a Tantric sādhana. In some traditions, they even rejoice at this moment because it means that the sādhana is doing its work: it is wringing us out. Or perhaps it is like a pimple or boil being brought to a head. It isn't pretty, but in the end it promotes healing and wholeness. It is part of the process of being in her fire for so long.

I share this with you so that you might exhale a little, perhaps, and feel yourself as part of this larger process. Please know that I am in it too, as is anyone who has also undertaken this sādhana commitment. Take a moment to feel into the web of connection you have established with Kālī, with me, and with all those who have committed to the practice of the *Song of the Hundred Names of Ādyā Kālī*, even if you don't know any of these people personally. We are all connected through the depth of sharing the same spiritual practice. You are not alone.

If this is a challenging moment for you, if unhealed aspects have surfaced, if you are in the shadow work, if you feel triggered, edgy, or re-traumatized, please give yourself the extra space and time and support you need to be with this and heal. Find a conversation partner, talk to your therapist, take long walks in nature, or slow baths. Journal, eat better than usual, and sleep more than usual. I also recommend Bach's Five-Flower Formula (akin to Rescue Remedy), and lots of warm water. Please find ways to reduce your stress levels, even if temporarily.

I urge you all to move into more subtle levels of self care that includes space and time for your personal process and healing. In addition, you might want to have a talk with Ādyā Kālī about what is happening for you, and ask for her support. Perhaps leave out extra offerings on your shrine. When you do the daily recitation of her names, dedicate the practice to your own healing, and the healing of the others with us in this sādhana. You may want to use the *klīṃ* bīja as a kind of protective mantra to help you through this moment as well. Her embodiment and protection and healing work are in the bīja, and in the recitation of her names.

96) Kāmabījasvarūpiṇī (She Who Is the Embodiment of the Bīja Mantra *Klīṃ*, She Who Is the Form of the Kāma Bīja)

Ādyā Kālī is the form of all things . . . can you sense this for yourself now that you have undergone your own direct experience? Can you feel this in your body somewhere? If so, where? She is also the form of the healing of that which is unhealed, as many of you know directly now. She brings forth the wounding, and is the healing. In the hottest parts of India, during the monsoon, they say that she gives the pox and takes it away, she gives the disease and she heals. So it is here. Know that what is happening for you is her sacred work. As I settle into that and surrender to that, my own healing unfolds with more grace and ease and far less anxiety. This is her work and we are in her lap.

The bīja mantra *klīṃ* has a sound, and that sound is her form; Kāmabījasvarūpiṇī-Kāmākhyā-Kālī's form is also the bīja mantra *klīṃ*. It is her and she is it. What is your own experience of potency of the bīja in this name? Can you feel in your body how she is the utterance of her bīja? *Klīṃ* is Kālī-Kāmākhyā; Kāmkhyā-Kālī is *klīṃ*.

Klīṃ is also one of the bīja associated with desire. Desire is the storehouse of śakti in the yoniverse. The vibration of the bīja on your lips and in your womb-pelvis and heart will activate the śakti that brings forth the healing energies you need right now. Desire is one of the forms of śakti, and śakti is just another way of describing the energies of love moving, just as Kālī is love in form.

May Kāmabījasvarūpiṇī-Kālī's bīja and śakti and love be with you during these last days.

97) Kumatighnī (She Who Is the Destroyer of all Evil Inclinations)

This is what we asked for; this is where we asked her to take us, even when we didn't know where we would end up. She is clearing out everything and anything that keeps you separate from her. Everything that is arising is the work of this sādhana. Can you keep going and let this finish? Kumatighnī-Kālī can take whatever is arising. Give it to her. It is all hers anyway.

Offer all the rough spots, the challenges, the edginess, the emotions, at her feet. Give it all to her. Pour it out to her. She is asking for it; she is waiting to receive all of what is moving through you. Give it to her as an offering at your shrine during your recitation. She will remove the darkness and difficulty. She will remove all you feel that might be called "evil." Set it down at her feet and be open to receive what she offers. Can you imagine this possibility? Can you open to this potential? Can you find your way in the dark back to her lotus feet, to her lap?

I offer my practice up to each of you who have made a practice commitment to the *Song of the Hundred Names of Ādyā Kālī*, and for the quick passage of all that is arising in this moment. I offer up my practice to your well being and healing and safety. I offer my practice up to your awakening, in this lifetime, in a female body, in a male body, in the body.

98) Kulīnārtināśinī (She Who Is the Destroyer of the Afflictions of the Kaulika)

What is there to say today that I haven't already said in this last run of her names? She has us in all this. Everything that she has given us, she takes back into herself. All the troubles, the turmoils, the challenges, the edginess, the fear, the anger, the shadows . . . She will destroy them all for us, as her devotees, as her children. Give them all to Kulīnārtināśinī today with your recitation. Offer her all the blessings and all the challenges. She will take them all into herself and transform them. Just as we take it all into ourselves and transform it. Allow this to unfold for you today. Allow softness and surrender and full self-love and self-acceptance to lead you. Kulīnārtināśinī-Kālī has our backs.

99) Kulakāminī (She Who Is the Entire Family of Desires, She Who Is the Lady of the Kula, the Kaula)

She is everything we want and need. She is our Lady. She is the one who loves us. She is our mother and we are her children. Kulakāminī encompasses us completely, and she is the form of every desire we have. She is the form of all that is related to our desire. Her desire is our desire. She is our mother and our family in this. With her, we are truly never alone. Kulakāminī-Kālī is the one who leads us to the end of the path that the Kaulas undertake. This is Kālī's path, and she will take us there. Let yourself fall into her sweet guidance and liberation today. Let yourself fall into her protection. Let yourself fall into her family, which is our family, our kula. Welcome home.

100) Kālakaṇṭakaghātinī (She Who Is by the Bīja, *Krīṃ, Hrīṃ, Śrīṃ*, the Destroyer of the Fear of Death)

As the liturgy concludes, "These are known as the Hundred Names of Devī Ādyā Kālikā, beginning with the letter KA. They are all identical with the form of Kālī." Jai Kālakaṇṭakaghātinī Mā, Jai! I rejoice. I feel bittersweet. I'm melancholy and I'm at peace. I am offering obeisance to her today as I write this contemplation. I have put out extra offerings and been on my knees. It seems that there is no other place to be right now except on my knees in gratitude. I also have a sense of soft humility; this is so much larger, more vast, more blissful, and more loving than I have ever known. This is so much bigger than me, or us, and I'm honored and grateful that her work is my offering to the world. I am her servant, there is no doubt.

When we consider the depths of our fear of death, we might begin to understand that the fear of death and associated loss is underneath almost all of our shadow and wounding. We are deeply afraid of death, most of us. We can see how Kālī's practices are meant to help us come to terms with this fear, and thus liberate us. When we are not large enough for this work, in any moment, we can always gaze upon her image, find her form, for what we need. Let me explain.

Did you know that Kālī's upper right hand is raised in what is known as the *abhaya* mudrā that indicates Kālī's neverending assertion to her children: "Fear not!" she says. She says it forever; she never stops saying it to us as reassurance and reminder. Kālī's lower right hand is an open palm with the fingers pointing to the earth: this is the offering of all that we desire. All that we need and want is drizzling off her fingertips towards us. Can we drink in her protection? Can we release our fears to her so there is room to drink in her blessings?

The bīja mantras *krīṃ, hrīṃ,* and *śrīṃ* are the sounds of creation, preservation, and transformation. The three sides of her yonic triangle. Through the cycle of these three bīja, Kālī Mā takes care of all the cycles of existence and all our needs. I do *not* recommend that you use these mantras though. These are her bīja and I would leave the power of these bīja to her, especially at times like this. Each of those bīja requires its own sādhana, commitment, and depth of practice. As you know by now, this is not to be undertaken lightly nor without guidance from a qualified gurvī or guru.

Today, please do dedicate your recitation of the liturgy and offer out the blessings of these 108 nights for the benefit of all beings. I am sending blessings and gratitude to each of you.

❀ ❀ ❀

Please take down your Ādyā Kālī shrine (for wandering yoginīs and yogis, please do this as soon as you return to your main shrine). It is important to bring the sādhana to a close by doing this. You may, of course, re-establish a new Kālī shrine for your regular practice life, or integrate Kālī into your other shrines. It is time for the shrine to change. This is important to do. I have had challenges when I didn't re-do the shrine at the end of a practice commitment, and I would love for all of you to have graceful ease at the end of this sādhana.

I send blessings and gratitude to each of you. *Jai Mā*!

Closing Prayers

ॐ ब्रह्मार्पणं ब्रह्म हविर्ब्रह्माग्नौ ब्रह्मणा हुतम्।
ब्रह्मैव तेन गन्तव्यं ब्रह्मकर्मसमाधिना।।

oṁ brahmārpaṇaṃ brahma havirbrahmāgnau brahmaṇā hutam |
brahmaiva tena gantavyaṃ brahmakarmasamādhinā | |

Oṁ [Kālī-] Brahman makes the offering; [Kālī-] Brahman is the offering; offered by [Kālī-] Brahman, in the fire of [Kālī-] Brahman. By seeing [Kālī-] Brahman in all actions, one realizes that [Kālī-] Brahman.

ॐ पूर्णमदः पूर्णमिदं पूर्णात् पूर्णमुदच्यते।
पूर्णस्य पूर्णमादाय पूर्णमेवावशिष्यते।।

oṁ pūrṇamadaḥ pūrṇamidaṃ pūrṇāt pūrṇamudacyate |
pūrṇasya pūrṇamādāya pūrṇamevāvaśiṣyate | |

Oṁ That is whole and perfect; this is whole and perfect. From the whole and perfect, the whole and perfect becomes manifest. If the whole and perfect issue forth from the whole and perfect, even still only the whole and perfect will remain.

क्षमास्व

kṣamāsya

Please forgive me [for any errors that I might have made in the offering of this *sādhana*]

oṁ karmaṇā manasā vācā tvatto nānya gatir mama ।
antaścāreṇa bhūtānāṁ draṣṭā tvaṁ parameśvari । ।

Oṁ With our actions, mind, and speech, we have no other goal than you, who by dwelling within, witnesses all beings, O Supreme Goddess.

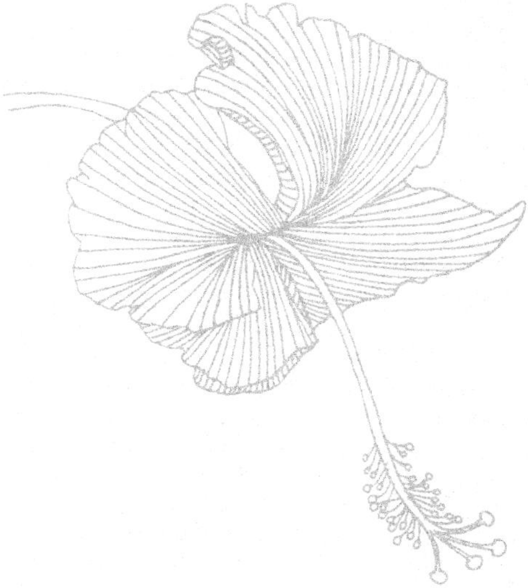

Acknowledgements

This is a full-bodied offering to the fierce dark Tantric goddess Kālī Mā and to my teachers, friends, beloveds, and family during this long and sublime journey. This is far more of a supported relationship-based collaborative undertaking than it might appear on first look. An entire community brought this book forth through their dedication, love, and practice. I have never been alone in this unfolding into Kālī's worlds even when I felt I was. A beloved sakhī was with me when I first met Kālī and relationship continues to be a primary part of this spiritual path. One of the fundamental aspects of this path of relationship with Kālī and the Kālīkula is devotion. Devotion cannot exist without relationship, relationship to oneself and to the lover and the beloved. Sometimes, it is our devotion that opens the door to relationship. Sometimes though, it is through relationship that we discover what we didn't even know we would become devoted to. From there, the power of desire emerges.

To those who are woven into the very womb-heart stream of my life, at different times, in different places, I offer my deepest gratitude and respect for the love, support, inspiration, guidance, and companionship. You are my kula, my paramparā. To the circle of practitioners, consummate lineage holders, women and men of love, women and men in love, let me name you for all that has flowed from you to me over the years in support of these practices coming to fruition. This nāmāvalī is a garland of gratitude for the precious jewels of deep enduring relationship; it starts at the beginning and moves towards today weaving together the deepest and most potent connections in my life that allowed this book to flow forth: Demi Russell, Byron Harlon, Suma Datta, Sindhu Nakarmi, the women on Lazimpat, Sheila and Narendra, Jenny Thomas, Andrew Manzardo, Sofia O. Diaz, Eduardo Pagán, Paul Kallmes, Chandra Alexandre, Kelley Lampiasi, Susan Burggraf, Penny Gill, Max Dashu, Herukala, Swamiji, Heather Roberts-McEvoy, Julia Vigdis Au-Perkins, Frédérique Apffel, Neela Bhattacharya Saxena, Asherah Allen, Laura Ambika Amazzone, April Heaslip, Davesh Soneji, the Swamis: Heidi and Mike, Lamala, Rinpochela, Sakhi Devi, Shyam, Renee Ryerson, Mary-Louise Walton, K.S., Shiva and Demetri, Sreedevi Bringi, Arwen, Christina, Willow Pearson, Birrell Walsh, Vamadeva, Justine Sanchez, Ara Lawton, Una Strauss, Regina Sara Ryan, Prem M., the dedicated yoginīs and yogis of the kula, Dawn Cartwright, Nisha Bhairavi, Vajra Ma, Geanna Gonzales-Wood, Dorothy Walters, the Goldman family (especially Ora), Sarita, and the following communities: Mount Holyoke College, Shannon Paige and Om Time Yoga, the Integral Center, and the Red Thread Collective. For support in the final preparation of this manuscript, I want to especially acknowledge Regina and Durgadasi Devi; your attention to detail with such love and devotion is the grace of hibiscus and jasmine at her feet. Citrajoyti rushed to bring the offerings of the illustrations to fruition, imbuing the book with auspicious grace and beauty. Shyam's last minute mantric sharing brought it all into union. All of you have encouraged me to go more deeply still, to offer it all, to be an offering, to offer what has been transmitted. You have called me into my own knowing and supported me there. I honor you. Because of you, I can do nothing but supplicate the inner ocean.

Many Tantric Śākta goddess communities in South Asia have shared their private sādhanas, teachings, transmissions, initiations, festivals, families, and homes with me over the years, including at Dakṣiṇkālī, Paśupatināth, Kāmākhyā, Jvālāmukhī, Kālīghāt and Dakṣiṇeśvar: in Kathmandu, Kolkata, Delhi, and the jungles of eastern India. This has not always been easy, or without consequence. Your courage and willingness to sit in circle with me for so long, to walk on pilgrimage, and to practice around the ancient fires is the blessing of my teachers and the teachings. Pranāms to the śaktis and the bhairavs, the yoginīs and vīras of the Śākta Pīṭha. There is no separation. Lineage and love flow because of you.

My blood family: I honor you deeply. You brought me into this world and showed me the path. I anoint your individual and collective feet for all that we have been through together. It has not been easy, I know. I love you still.

This book is dedicated to the fullest garland of beloveds: my mother (mamala), my teachers (gurvīs and gurus), my sakhī, bhairavs, and my students. The Yoginīs open the gate, the Ḍākinīs whisper, and thus lineage flows from the mouths, body to body, all as one. No one left behind. To the unnamed and undocumented yoginīs and yogis of South Asia who led the way in their fierce, glorious, unfettered, and disciplined ways: there are no words that express what you offer us on the path.

Endnotes

Every effort has been made to trace copyright holders of material in this book. The author and editors apologize if any work has been used without permission, and would be glad to be told of anyone who has not been consulted.

Introduction

1 Used with permission. www.yogawithina.com.

2 क

3 See the Bibliography for a full list of Sanskrit language and English language sources for the *Song of the Hundred Names of Ādyā Kālī* from the *Mahānirvāna Tantra*.

4 I use standard diacritics for Indic languages in this book because they offer precision in terminology and naming. As your studies and devotion deepen, the scented trail of precise spelling and accurate terminology will unfold towards the original sources themselves. I do not want to gloss over this, as the sādhana is in the details. When quoting from other sources and translations, I follow the use of diacritics as found in those sources.

5 Used with permission.

6 "Archean" refers a time period that extends from the origin of the earth to 2,500 million years ago; the origin and the way back old school.

7 For more on Lajjāgaurī, see Bapat (2008) and Bolon (1992).

8 From the *Bhairava Yamala*: translation from *Light of Consciouness Journal* (Truth Consciousness), spring 2008, p. 80. Used with permission.

9 For more on Dakṣiṇeśwar Kālī and her temple, see Harding (1993).

10 One version of the story can be found at http://www.adyapeath.org/Story.html (accessed April 7, 2013). For more on the life and teachings of Rāmakṛṣṇa and Śrī Śāradā Devī see Harding (1993) and Olson (1990).

11 I might go so far as to say, in a low voice, that Ādyā Pīṭh is an ultimate reality consort shrine.

12 Some other details to help fill out your understanding of Ādyā Kālī as part of this non-random love-matrix yoniverse has to do with a further unfolding of the term *ādyā*. For example, *ādyā śakti* is one of the terms for a female consort and she is the primordial *śakti* in union with us at all times.

13 These are names 22 and 25 in the *Song*. Please see the Contemplations for more details on the dark as they relate to these individual names.

14 Inanna's descent to the underworld is detailed in Diane Wolkstein's book *Inanna: Queen of Heaven and Earth* (1983).

15 "Moon blood" is another term for menstrual blood.

16 For more on Śaivism, see Müller-Ortega (1989).

17 June McDaniel has also made this same distinction of the forms of Śāktism in contemporary South Asia (2004:4ff).

18 Indeed, there are even Śākta goddesses who emanate as the sixteen phases of the moon: the Nityās. For more on the Kālī Nityās, see http://www.shivashakti.com/kali3.htm. For more on the Lalitā Nityās, see http://www.shivashakti.com/nitya.htm.

19 The term *kula* refers to a *clan* or Tantric family. Here, we have the clan, or *kula*, of the goddess Śrī, the Śrīkula, and the clan or kula of Kālī, the Kālīkula.

20 To discover more about the south Indian Śrīvidyā lineages and their goddesses, see Brooks (1990, 1996).

21 For more on the Daśa Mahāvidyā, see Kinsley (1998), Frawley (1999), and my forthcoming book *The Yoginī's Womb*.

22 For more on the Mātṛkā, see Harper (1989), Aryan (1980), Panikkar (1997), and my forthcoming book *The Yoginī's Womb*.

23 For more on the Śākta Pīṭha, see Sircar (1978), Kinsley (1988) and my forthcoming book *The Yoginī's Womb*.

24 Another related and relevant term that you may come across is *kaula* which refers to the path itself, the specific practices, i.e. the Kaula Path, also referred to as Left-Handed Tantra.

25 The entire thought bears including here, in the treasure of footnotes: "This dual cosmogony represents a holistic feminine union, whereby the feminine twins can be seen as lovers, as mothers, as sisters, etc. In these early feminine cosmogonies one does not find consorted deities in a heterosexual arrangement, but dual deities of the same sex, referred to often as twins (*jami*). The union that is symbolized is neither static nor a complete merger but instead a coming together, a meeting out of movement" (Thadani 1996:21).

26 See Thadani (1996), especially Chapter Two on the Dual Feminine.

27 The practices and beliefs inherent in Śāktism continue to help us refine our assumptions of Hinduisms as universally oppressive to women, and help us to counteract the prevalent worldviews focused on unchanging hierarchies that place men over women and high-castes over low-castes. The kind of empowerment that many South Asian and western women experience as result of their devotion to the Śākta goddesses is, of course, not universal. We know the reality of South Asia women who lead difficult lives, even in

areas heavily entrenched in goddess worship. What it does mean though, is that for those of us looking for the interrelationships among the potent and powerful multiplicity of the divine feminine in our lives, there are practices, perspectives, and lineages that devotees can draw upon that foster both social empowerment and spiritual development.

28 For a general introduction to goddess worship in South Asia see Hawley and Wulff (1986), Kinsley (1988, 1989), and Kempton (2012).

29 For more on the distinction between independent goddesses and spousified goddesses see Gatwood (1985).

30 Tantric Buddhism is also known as either Vajrayana or Tibetan Buddhism.

31 For an in-depth analysis of the changing nature of Tantra and its relationship to western worlds, see McDermott and Kripal (2003) and Urban (2003).

32 *Kaula* is another term for those who worship Śakti in the left-handed Tantric paths.

33 *antah kaula bahiḥ śaivo janamadhye tu vaiṣḥavah* | | (*Kulārṇavatantra* 11.83) (Gupta 2012:393).

34 The *Śaktisaṃgama Tantra* is commonly dated from between the 6th to 8th centuries C.E.

35 For more on the Mahāvidyā, see Frawley (1999) and Kinsley (1998), and my forthcoming book, *The Yoginī's Womb.*

36 The lists of Mahāvidyās vary regionally and by lineage. As far as I have been able to ascertain, Kālī is the first of all the Mahāvidyās no matter the location, lineage, practice, or associated texts.

37 Kāmākhyā is the main deity at the center of my spiritual lineage and her temple in Assam is one of my spiritual homes.

38 For more on the relationship among the Śākta Pīṭha, the Mahāvidyā and Kāmākhyā, see my forthcoming book, *The Yoginī's Womb.*

39 Thus far, the *Bṛhannīla Tantra* has not been translated fully into English. A translation of Chapter 23 by Mike Magee includes the *Hundred Names of Kālī,* and can be found at http://www.sivaśakti.com/nila.htm. Magee refers to this text as the *Brihadnila Tantra.* A long synopsis of the *Bṛhannīla Tantra* can be found in Loriliai Biernacki's excellent book *Renowned Goddess of Desire* (2007:193-221).

40 The dating of Tantric texts is challenging at best. Biernacki dates the *Bṛhannīla Tantra* to the very late 1500s C.E. or early 1600s C.E. (2007:158). The *Mahānirvāna Tantra* is overall a much more conservative Tantra in terms of it's views of women and it is usually dated much later, perhaps as late as the 1800s C.E. although there are reasons to believe that it has an older form as well (Bhattacharyya 1999:84).

41 An early *Kālī Tantra* that elucidates this understanding is the *Kāmadhenutantra* dating from around the 16th century and originating from Bengal (Goudriaan 1981:83).

42 According to scholar and translator, Mike Magee: "Strictly speaking, a Yāmala is a different class of text, and supposed to pre-date the Tantras. However,

manuscripts of the Yāmala seem to be lost, except as quotations in later works." (http://www.shivashakti.com/rudrayam.htm, accessed 1/19/2013)

43 According to scholars, only one copy of the manuscript seems to have survived and is in the library of the Royal Asiatic Society of Bengal in Kolkata. This text contains approximately 550 *ślokas*, or syllabic verses (Goudriaan 1981:76). I had the honor of viewing this unique manuscript in the summer of 2013.

44 A *paramparā* is a spiritual family, a group of people who are "related" through Tantric spiritual practices, teachings, and teachers. This may or may not overlap with a blood family, a family of kin, the social family that is a *parivār* or *pariwār* (Hindi, Assamese, Nepali). These distinctions can sometimes be confusing since a paramparā will use kinship terms in much the same way that a pariwār does. How this unfolds in daily life and how this is represented in the Tantric literature is one of the ancient mysteries.

45 Along with my earlier scholarly work, anthropologist Sarah Caldwell describes the living allegory for Śāktas among women, the earth, and the goddess in Kerala (1999: 113). To offer you a taste of how this might look, on the ground, Caldwell writes:

> Because the earth is itself a divine female being, infused with life-force or sakti, the portrayal of the earth's phases in terms of the fertility of women is more than a metaphor. It is a living allegory, a visible expression of a known truth about the fundamental interconnection between all forms of life. Just as the goddesses divine power can move freely and without changing its essential nature from a statue to a tree to a lamp to a drawing and from there into the person of a possessed actor, in the same the dancing Bhagavati of muttiyettu does not *symbolize* the agricultural landscape but simply is that landscape expressing itself in a different form (1999:132).

46 We don't focus on the transmission of *śaktipāt* (or kuṇḍalinī) in my lineage as this energy is understood to arise naturally as a result of the other spiritual practices that we undertake: No special transmission or instruction is needed.

47 Source unknown.

48 Please see the Contemplations for more on the mysteries of these *bīja*.

49 Please see the Contemplations for more details on how this works specifically in the context of a recitation of the *Song of the Hundred Names of Adyā Kālī*.

50 You can find these small metal yantras on eBay and other online sites. Please be very careful about purchasing these from vendors that you don't know. Many of the ones that I've seen are improperly labeled and the actual etched yantra is not a form of the deity that corresponds with the northern Kālīkula forms. If you have any questions, do try to have someone you trust look at it for you before purchasing. It's also perfect to use the simpler method of laying out uncooked rice or flower petals under the yoni pot.

Another caveat about buying a metal yantra online is that some vendors are actually priests or ashrams and they may bless or consecrate the yantra before sending it to you. I prefer an unconsecrated yantra that I can charge with the specific energies that are in alignment with my relationship to Kālī.

You may be able to ask an online vendor to *not* consecrate it before sending it to you and then charge it with the energies of your shrine, practice, and devotion. Let your direct relationship with Kālī guide you here.

Song of the Hundred Names of Ādyā Kālī

1 Ganjā berries are the red and black berries used as weights by goldsmiths.

Contemplations of Ādyā Kālī's Hundred Names

1 The lives of Tantric female spiritual practitioners are not as well known as the lives of the male Tantrics. You can find some details of these women and their accomplishments online, and scattered here and there. I aspire to come out with a collection of the stories of some of these women before too long.

2 Used with permission.

3 *Immergence*: to submerge or disappear in, or as if in, liquid [archaic].

Glossary

abhaya mudrā	The hand gesture, mudrā, that signifies fearlessness; a gesture from the deity to the devotee that communicates "fear not."
Ambuvācī	The annual menstrual festival for the Goddess, earth, and women in Assam and other parts of eastern India.
amṛta	Tantric nectar, divine ambrosia.
añjali mudrā	The lotus mudrā; the palms are pressed together in front of the heart. This is a gesture of greeting as well as prayer and invocation.
āsana yoga	Literally: *seat*. This is the seat one takes for meditation or a yogic posture, as in the practice of Hatha yoga. It can also mean a bodily posture, or to come into the posture that one takes for sādhana.
bījā mantra	The term *bīja mantra* can be translated as either "essence mantra" or "seed mantra." These powerful single syllable sounds are called "seed mantras" because they contain the entire potentiality of the deity in much the same way that a seed holds the entire potential for a tree. Thus, the mantra is the deity, in entirety.

bindu	Literally, *drop, point,* or *center.* The term has cosmic philosophical significance as it indicates the dense energetic pulsing of the center of a yantra. A bindu is dynamic, multidimensional, and has its own properties. The sacred dynamic center point of a sacred diagram, cosmology, or geographic. The bindu is the densification of śakti before manifestation and after destruction, in the cosmic cycle. Form emerges from the bindu and dissolves back into it. See *tīlaka.*
brahman	Ultimate nondual reality; union. Also called kālibrahman.
cakra	A wheel or circle; one of the many circular energy centers in the body; sometimes used interchangeably with *maṇḍala*; the discus carried by Viṣṇu.
darśan	Literally, seeing or viewing; a way of coming into sensory contact with the divine.
Daśa Mahāvidyā	The Ten Wisdom Goddesses. A group of Hindu Tantric Goddesses who find their home on the Kāmākhyā temple hill, as well as at other Śākta Tantra Goddess Temples.
Devī	Goddess.
dhyāna	The term for a visualization of the deity used during meditation. It also refers to the unbroken riverine concentration found during meditation.
ghāt	A place, usually on the banks of a river, where bodies are cremated.

Gopī	Rādhā's female companions in mainstream Hinduism. The term *Gopī* emanates from the world of Rādhā and Kṛṣṇa. Rādhā's best friends, the milk-maid gopīs, are also referred to as the *sakhī*. Kṛṣṇa is not only Rādhā's beloved, but also the beloved of each and every Gopī. The Gopī are the ones who dress Rādhā to meet Kṛṣṇa and receive her when she returns, just as our sakhī do for us when union with our beloved is in the air. Rādhā's sakhī, the Gopī, are as much a part of Rādhā's world as Kṛṣṇa. Here, the term *Gopī* refers to the yoginīs who inhabit the forest of desire, and who are our spiritual sisters and support on the path. The Gopī are mature female practitioners living as householders who belong to a sacred community of other female practitioners. The Gopī are our sakhī.
guru	A qualified male spiritual teacher. See *gurvī*.
gurvī	A qualified female spiritual teacher, a female guru. See *guru*.
iṣṭadevatā	The chosen deity (masculine). See *iṣṭadevī*.
iṣṭadevī	The chosen deity (feminine). See *iṣṭadevatā*.
jami	A philosophical principle of feminine twinship, feminine duality that comprises a whole. The union of the dual feminine.
japa	The spiritual practice of reciting a mantra using a mālā to count the repetitions.
Kālīkula	One of the major wisdom streams of Śāktism, and the focus of this book. A north Indian Tantric goddess worship associated with all the forms and energies of the dark moon, known

as the Kālīkula. The Kālīkula focuses on the dark goddess Kālī and the other groups of goddesses that emanate from her and are her wisdom manifest. The goddesses include Kālī (in all her forms), the Daśa Mahāvidyā (the Ten Great Wisdoms), the Mātṛkā (the Mothers), and the other goddesses associated with Satī's body parts at the *Śākta Pīṭha.* The Kālīkula is geographically centered in, but not limited to, Assam, Bihar, Orissa, West Bengal, Bangladesh, as well as parts of Maharashtra.

kāma	*Kāma* is the Sanskrit term for "desire."
kapāla	A Tantric ritual implement; a drinking vessel made from a human skull; a skull cup.
kaula	A term for those whose practice the left-handed forms of Śākta Tantra.
kula	The term *kula* refers to a *clan* or tantric family. For example, we have the clan, or kula, of the goddess Śrī, the Śrīkula, and the clan or kula of Kālī, the Kālīkula. A kula is different from a tantric lineage, or *paramparā,* in that the *kula* is widespread and not all members will share practices, teachings, teachers or beliefs. A *kula* is more horizontal and wide-spread in nature, even though hierarchies certainly do exist. See *paramparā.*
kulācāra	The teachings of the kula, the way of those who belong to the kula, the left-handed Tantric path of the kula practitioner.
Kumarī	Pre-menarchal girls understood to be embodiments of the goddess. To please or worship a Kumarī is to please or worship Devī.

līlā	The cosmic "play" of the goddesses and gods, usually with specific reference to the play of Rādhā and Kṛṣṇa, and the Gopī. It can also refer to the cosmic play of the universe.
liṅga	The male generative organ; the cosmic phallus; a phallus; synonymous with Śiva. A symbol of divine creation when associated with the *yoni*.
makāra	Aka *pañcamakāra*; the five sacred Tantric feast offerings.
mālā	A rosary used to count mantra recitations. See *japa*.
maṇḍala	A complex two- or three-dimensional geometrical diagram used in ritual and meditative practices. The home, or palace, of the deity. The term maṇḍala is usually, but not always, associated with Tantric Buddhist practices. They are also called *yantras* in some cultural contexts. See *yantra*.
Mātṛkā	A group of seven or eight Tantric goddesses, the Mothers, who encircle the outer edges of the landscape.
mudrā	A physical gesture used in ritual contexts that invokes and moves specific energies for specific purposes, normally inside of a sādhana or other ritual practice. Sometimes the term mudrā is translated as "seal" pointing to how a mudrā can be used to "seal" energy into a particular place or form. Mudrās are a tangible way of bringing energies into form and to enhance our embodiment of those energies.

mūrti — A consecrated statue of the deity used in worship. It also means "embodiment" or "figure."

paramparā — A paramparā is a spiritual family based in lineage. Paramparā are sometimes even centered in family households. A paramparā is more intimate than a kula, and will share a common ancestor, teachers, and teachings. A paramparā may have a lineage-descent structure, with unique practices and teachings coming down from a gurvī or guru. See *kula*.

pīṭha — The sacred seat, or location, of a goddess. The sacred place where a goddess is enthroned in her temple; a central location for the worship of the deity. See *śākta pīṭha*.

praṇām mantra — These are longer forms of mantras that usually end with the words *svāhā* or *namaḥ*. A praṇām mantra offers homage, praise, and supplication to the deity. They can be used to begin to approach the deity.

pūjā — An expression of honor and respect through ritual; a form of worship and devotion.

rūpā — Form, or embodied form. The form that existence takes. The form that a deity takes.

sādhana — Spiritual discipline; a formal spiritual practice within a lineage. The term can refer to the liturgy itself, or the spiritual practice, or both.

sakhī — The term *sakhī* refers to one's most intimate girlfriends, the ones on the inside, the inner circle. Our sakhī share our practices with us, who are in the yoginī cakra, who know that Kālī and union are the center of the yoniverse. The term *sakhī* emanates from the world of Rādhā and Kṛṣṇa. Rādhā's best friends, the milk-maid Gopī, are also referred to as the sakhī. Kṛṣṇa is not only Rādhā's beloved, but also the beloved of each and every Gopī. The Gopī are the ones who dress Rādhā to meet Kṛṣṇa and receive her when she returns, just as our sakhī do for us when union with our beloved is in the air. Rādhā's sakhī, the Gopī, are as much a part of Rādhā's world as Kṛṣṇa. Sakhī is a term of intimate sisterhood, in community.

Śaivism — One of the major forms of Tantric Hinduism that focuses on Śiva as ultimate nondual reality.

Śaivite — Someone who practices Śaivism.

Śākta — Refers to a specific stream of tantric Hinduism where the goddess is the central deity. Also, someone who practices Śākta Tantra; a devotee of the Śākta Goddesses.

Śākta Pīṭha — The sacred seat, or location, of a Tantric Śākta goddess. The sacred place where a goddess is enthroned in her temple; a central location for the worship of the Śākta goddess. Sometimes used to refer to the places in the Indic landscape where the different parts of the goddess' body parts fell, according to one myth.

Śakti — Śakti, as a proper noun (capitalized, without italics), refers to goddess, the goddess, in her undifferentiated form, before she separates into her constituent parts. Śakti is identical to the Great Mother, Devī, Kālī, Ādyā Kālī, and is the lifeblood energy of creation. She is an independent goddess, whole unto herself and

	simultaneously part of everything, imbued with everything.
śakti	The Sanskrit root of *śakti* is *śak*, meaning "potency," "the potential to produce," "to be able," "to do," or "to act." Śakti refers to "primordial energy, the source of all divine and cosmic evolution" (Bhattacharyya 2002:139). Part of this energetic relationality is that śakti is personified in all the forms we find in the natural world; it is the energy that animates all life.
sandhyā bhāṣā	The coded Tantric twilight language that is used in Tantric texts and practices.
saṅkalpa	A vow, or commitment, to undertake a spiritual practice or sādhana. It implies intention and resolve to complete the sādhana.
seva	Selfless service, work done without attachment to one's own benefit.
siddhi	The term for spritual attainment in the Tantric lineages.
sindūr	The red ritual powder used to mark the forehead, the third eye, as well as to annoint statues. See *tīlaka* and *bindu*.
Śrīvidyā	One of the forms of Śāktism that focuses on the goddess Śrī (aka Tripurā Sundarī).
stotra	Or *stotram*; a Sanskrit hymn to a deity.
tattva	One way that the term *tattva* can be translated is as *fundamental*; and in this system, there are at least thirty-six fundamental building blocks of manifest existence. Kālī is here in the tattvas,

	linking them all together in her body. A tattva is an *element* or aspect of manifest existence that comes forth from the formless deity into concrete manifestation. Examples of tattvas in manifestation include earth, water, fire, air, ether, what we know as the senses (the mediums for olfactory sensations, taste sensations, visual sensations, etc.), excretion, sexuality, movement, apprehension/understanding, speech; locomotion is her tattva too.
tīlaka	A sacred mark on the forehead between the eyebrows that often signifies that one has had darśan or undertaken pūjā. Sometimes the style of the tīlaka signifies association with a particular spiritual lineage or sect or worshipped deity. The mark can also be for beautification or medicinal reasons. See *bindu*.
ugrā	Ugrā is variously translated as *powerful, mighty, strong, violent, terrible, fierce, cruel, ferocious, hot* and *sharp*.
Vaiṣṇava	Someone who practices Vaiṣṇavism.
Vaiṣṇavism	A form of Hinduism where Viṣṇu is understood as the supreme deity, ultimate reality.
varṇa mālā	The string of letters that comprise the Sanskrit alphabet. Literally, the mālā of the letters or syllables of the alphabet.
vrata	A *vrata* is a commitment to spiritual practice (like the sādhana of reciting her names) in order to achieve blessings of one's desires as well as to mature in our spiritual awareness, moving ever more dynamically into union with full embodied awakening. Technically, *vrata* means

to vow or *promise*. The term *vrata* also sometimes carries the taste of making a sacrifice or promise to the goddess in order to achieve one's aims.

yantra — A sacred two- or three-dimensional geometric diagram used in meditative and ritual practices. The home, or palace, of the deity, as well as the unfolding of the mystery of the deity. In some contexts, the terms *yantra* and *maṇḍala* are used interchangeably. See *maṇḍala*.

yoni — The Sanskrit word *yoni* has multiple layers of meaning, as is common in tantric practices. Some of the translations include 1. womb, vulva, vagina; 2. place of birth, source, origin, spring; 3. abode, home, lair, nest; or 4. family, race, stock, caste, etc. The word *yoni* is etymologically derived from the Sanskrit root *yuj* meaning to "join," "unite," "fasten," or "harness." (Apffel-Marglin 1987). This is the same root for the word *yoga*, which I often translate as "the art of moving into union." Thus, the yoni can be understood as that which is joining or uniting. It is active, almost an action, or activity.

yoni-maṇḍala — Synonymous with *yoni-yantra*; the array of the yoni, into all of it's mandalic display. The maṇḍala of the yoni; the yoni as a maṇḍala.

yoni-mudrā — The mudrā of the yoni; the hand gesture used in ritual and meditative practices to signify the yoni.

yoni-pīṭha — From a Śakta point of view, this is a sacred place of the yoni of the goddess; an established place where the yoni of the goddess is worshipped.

yoni-yantra — Synonymous with *yoni-maṇḍala*; the array of the yoni, into all of it's mandalic display. The yantra that is the yoni; the yoni as a yantra.

Bibliography

Anonymous

2008 Excerpt from the *Bhairava Yamala*. *Light of Consciouness Journal* (Truth Consciousness) spring:80.

Apffel-Marglin, Frédérique

1987 "Yoni." *The Encyclopedia of Religion*. Mircea Eliade, editor. Volume 15. Pp. 530-535. New York: Macmillam Publishing Company.

Aryan, K. C.

1980 *The Little Goddesses (Mātrikās)*. New Delhi: Rekha Prakashan.

Avalon, Arthur (aka Sir John Woodroffe) and Ellen Avalon

1964 *Hymns to the Goddess*. Translated from the Sanskrit. Madras: Ganesh and Company.

Bapta, Jayant Bhalchandra

2008 "The Lajjāgaurī: Mother, Wife or Yoginī." *The Iconic Female: Goddesses of India, Nepal and Tibet*. Jayant Bhalchandra Bapat and Ian Mabbett, editors. Pp. 79-111. Clayton: Monash University Press.

Barks, Coleman, translator

1992 *Naked Song: Lalla*. Athens, GA: Maypop Books.

Bhattacharyya, N. N. [Narendra Nath]

2002 *Tantrābhidhāna: A Tantric Lexicon*. Delhi: Manohar.

Biernacki, Loriliai

2007 *Renowned Goddess of Desire: Women, Sex and Speech in Tantra*. Oxford University Press.

Bolon, Carol Radcliffe

1992 *Forms of the Goddess Lajjā Gaurī in Indian Art*. Delhi: Motilal Banarsidass Publishers.

Brooks, Douglas Renfew
1996 *Auspicious Wisdom: The Texts and Traditions of Śrīvidyā Śākta Tantrism in South India.* New Delhi: Manohar Publishers.

1990 *The Secret of the Three Cities: An Introduction to Hindu Śākta Tantra.* Chicago: Chicago University Press.

Caldwell, Sarah
1999 *Oh Terrifying Mother: Sexuality, Violence and the Worship of the Goddess Kālī.* New Delhi: Oxford University Press/Oxford India Paperbacks.

Chitgopekar, Nilima
2002 "The Unfettered Yoginīs." *Invoking Goddesses: Gender Politics in Indian Religion.* Nilima Chitgopekar, editor. Pp. 82-111. Delhi: Shakti Books (An Imprint of Har-Anand Publications Pvt Ltd).

Dehejia, Vidya
1986 *Yogini Cult and Temples: A Tantric Tradition.* New Delhi: National Museum.

Dutt, M.N., translator, and J.L. Gupta, editor
2010 *Mahānirvāṇatantraṃ: Sanskrit Text, Transliteration and English Translation with Copious Notes.* Varanasi: Chowkhamba Vidyabhawan.

Frawley, David
1999 *Tantric Yoga and the Wisdom Goddesses: Spiritual Secrets of Ayurveda.* Delhi: Motilal Banarsidass Publishers.

Gadon, Elinor
2002 "Probing the Mysteries of the Hirapur Yoginis." *ReVision* 25(1):33-41.

Gatwood, Lynn E.
1985 *Devī and the Spouse Goddess: Women, Sexuality, and Marriages in India.* Riverdale, MD: The Riverdale Company.

Goudriaan, Teun
1981 "Chapter IV: Tantras Devoted to Kālī and Some Other Goddesses." *History of Indian Literature, Vol. 2: Hindu Tantric and Śākta Literature* by Teun Goudriaan and Sanjukta Gupta. Pp. 75-91. Wiesbaden: Otto Harrassowitz.

Gupta, Sanjukta Gombrich
2012 "Women in the Śaiva/Śākta Ethos." *The Cosmic Play of Power: Goddess, Tantra and Women*. Pp. 378-400. Delhi: Motilal Banarsidass Publishers.

Harding, Elizabeth Usha
1993 *Kali: The Black Goddess of Dakshineswar*. York Beach, ME: Nicolas-Hays Inc.

Harper, Katherine Anne
1989 *Seven Hindu Goddesses of Spiritual Transformation: The Iconography of the Saptamatrikas*. Lewiston, NY: Edwin Mellen Press.

Hawley, John Stratton and Donna Marie Wulff, editors
1986 *The Divine Consort: Radha and the Goddesses of India*. Boston: Beacon Press.

Kaimal, Padma
2002 "Tantra and the Kailāsanāth Temple in Kāñcīpuram." Paper presented at the 31st Annual Conference on South Asia, Madison, WI.

Kempton, Sally
2013 *Awakening Shakti: The Transformative Power of the Goddesses of Yoga*. Boulder, CO: Sounds True.

Kinsley, David
1998 *Tantric Visions of the Divine Feminine: The Ten Mahāvidyās*. Delhi: Motilal Banarsidass Publishers.

1989 *The Goddesses' Mirror: Visions of the Divine from East and West*. Albany, NY: State University of New York Press.

1988 *Hindu Goddesses: Vision of the Divine Feminine in the Hindu Religious Tradition*. Delhi: Motilal Banarsidass Publishers.

McDaniel, June
2004 *Offering Flowers and Feeding Skulls: Popular Goddess Worship in West Bengal*. Oxford and New York: Oxford University Press.

McDermott, Rachel Fell
2001 *Singing to the Goddess: Poems to Kali and Uma from Bengal*. Oxford and New York: Oxford University Press.

McDermott, Rachel Fell and Jeffrey J. Kripal, editors
2003 *Encountering Kali in the Margins, at the Center, in the West.* Berkeley, CA: University of California Press.

Müller-Ortega, Paul Eduardo
1989 *The Triadic Heart of Śiva: Kaula Tantricism of Abhinavagupta in the Non-Dual Shaivism of Kashmir.* Albany, NY: State University of New York Press.

Nathan, Leonard and Clinton Seely, translators
1999 *Grace and Mercy in Her Wild Hair: Selected Poems to the Mother Goddess by Rāmprasād Sen.* Prescott, AZ: HOHM Press.

Olson, Carl
1990 *The Mysterious Play of Kālī: An Interpretive Study of Rāmakrishna.* American Academy of Religion, Studies in Religion, Number 56. Atlanta, GA: Scholars Press.

Panikkar, Shivaji K.
1997 *Sapta Mātṛkā: Worship and Sculptures. An Iconological Interpretation of Conflicts and Resolutions in the Storied Brahmanical Icons.* Perspectives in Indian Art & Archaeology, no. 3. New Delhi: D. K. Printworld.

Rodrigues, Hillary Peter
2003 *Ritual Worship of the Great Goddess: The Liturgy of the Durgā Pūjā with Interpretations.* Albany, NY: State University of New York Press.

Saxena, Neela Bhattacharya
2004 *In the Beginning IS Desire: Tracing Kali's Footprints in Indian Literature.* New Delhi: Indialog.

Schelling, Andrew, editor
2011 *The Oxford Anthology of Bhakti Literature.* New Delhi: Oxford University Press.

Shaw, Miranda
1994 *Passionate Enlightenment: Women in Tantric Buddhism.* Princeton, NJ: Princeton University Press.

Sircar, D. C. [Dinesh Chandra]
1978 *The Śākta Pīṭhas.* Delhi: Motilal Banarsidas.

Thadani, Giti
1996 *Sakhiyani: Lesbian Desire in Ancient and Modern India*. London: Cassell.

Urban, Hugh B.
2003 *Tantra: Sex, Secrecy, Politics, and Power in the Study of Religion*. Berkeley, CA: University of California Press.

White, David Gordon
2003 *Kiss of the Yoginī: "Tantric Sex" in its South Asian Contexts*. Chicago: University of Chicago Press.

Wolkstein, Diane and Samuel Noah Kramer
1983 *Inanna: Queen of Heaven and Earth*. San Francisco: Harper and Row.

Additional Sources for

The *Song of the Hundred Names of Ādyā Kālī*

Avalon, Arthur (aka Sir John Woodroffe), editor, with the commentary of Hariharananda Bharati
2004 *Mahānirvāna Tantra*. Chapter Seven. Original publication in 1929. Delhi: Motilal Banarsidass. This version is in Sanskrit only with Sanskrit Commentary.

Avalon, Arthur (aka Sir John Woodroffe) and Ellen Avalon
1964 "Ādyākāli." *Hymns to the Goddess*. Translated from the Sanskrit. Pp. 40-48. Madras: Ganesh and Company.
This has the English translation in the main text and the names in English in the footnotes. No Sanskrit.

Douglas, Nik and Penny Slinger
nd "Adyakali Svarupa Stotra." http://yoniversum.nl/daktexts/kalistotra.html.
This is a list of the names in English with an English translation without intro or closing paragraphs. No Sanskrit. Accessed 8/22/2012.

Dutt, M.N., translator, and J.L. Gupta, editor
2010 *Mahānirvāṇatantram: Sanskrit Text, Transliteration and English Translation with Copious Notes*. Varanasi: Chowkhamba Vidyabhawan.

Rawson, Philip

1978 *The Art of Tantra*. Pp. 124-130. New York, NY: Thames and Hudson, Inc.

This is a unique and moving version that is an English-only translation and rendition without the introductory or final paragraphs. There is no numbering of either the names nor the paragraphs.

Saraswati, Swami Satyananda

1998 *Kālī Pūjā*. Third Edition. Pp. 92-111. Napa, CA: Devi Mandir Publications.

This is one of the fullest versions available and includes the original Sanskrit, Roman transliteration, as well as an English translation of the names, introductory paragraphs, and final paragraphs. This has unique *stotra* numbers.

Saraswati, Swami Bhajanananda

2006 *Kali Shata Nama: The Hundred Names of Goddess Kali*. Laguna Beach, CA: Kali Mandir.

This is a beautiful prayer booklet from the lineage of the esteemed teacher and Kālī devotee, Ramakrishna of Kolkata (Bhagavan Sri Ramakrishna Paramahamsa, 1836-1886 C.E.). This portable prayer book was designed so that devotees might carry it with them for personal practice. Portions of the original opening and concluding paragraphs are in the left margin as well as short explanations and teachings. It contains the Roman transliteration as well as English translation. This prayer book also includes a version of the names to be used as a *nāmāvalī* and a guide to pronunciation of the Sanskrit. The names are numbered, but there are no *stotra* numbers.

List of Illustrations

Every effort has been made to trace copyright holders of material in this book. The author and editors apologize if any work has been used without permission, and would be glad to be told of anyone who has not been consulted.

p. ii — Ādyā Kālī astride Śiva. Vintage tourist photograph. Private collection. Used with permission.

p. v — Gaṇeśa. Black and white illustration by Elke Citrajyoti Avis, 2013. Used with permission. http://iconsofessence.com and "Icons of Essence" on FaceBook.

p. vi — Śiva, Kālī, and the Mahāvidyā. Black and white illustration by Elke Citrajyoti Avis, 2013. Used with permission. http://iconsofessence.com and "Icons of Essence" on FaceBook.

p. 13 — Kālī Yoni Yantra. Black and white rendering of original cut paper art by Durgadasi Devi, 2012. Private collection. Used with permission.

p. 28 — The Face of Transformation: Kālī. Black and white illustration by Elke Citrajyoti Avis, 2013. Used with permission. http://iconsofessence.com and "Icons of Essence" on FaceBook.

p. 55 — *Jekhane Kālī, Sekhane Śiva.* Kālī. Black and white illustration by Elke Citrajyoti Avis, 2013. Used with permission. http://iconsofessence.com and "Icons of Essence" on FaceBook.

p. 74 — Womb Pot Preparation. Black and white rendering of color photograph, 2012. Private collection. Used with permission.

p. 75 Yoni Mudrā. Black and white illustration by Elke Citrajyoti Avis, 2013. Used with permission. http://iconsofessence.com and "Icons of Essence" on FaceBook.

p. 143 Abhaya Mudrā. Black and white illustration by Elke Citrajyoti Avis, 2013. Used with permission. http://iconsofessence.com and "Icons of Essence" on FaceBook.

Color Photo Credits

1 Kālī of the Cremation Grounds, Bakeshwar, West Bengal, 2011. Photograph by William Clark, www.kalibhakti.com. Used with permission. Associated with poem that starts at the bottom of p. 8.

2 Kālī Yoni Yantra. Cut paper art by Durgadasi Devi, 2012. Private collection. Used with permission. Associated with poem on p. 10.

3 One of the forms of Lajjāgaurī, the squatting Goddess menstruating, adorning the outside walls of the Kāmākhyā Temple in Assam, India. Photograph by the author, 2013. Associated with description on p. 13.

4 An open air round tree shrine to Bhairavī Brāmaṇī (aka Yogesvarī), one of Rāmakṛṣṇa's most important teachers, a Tantric yoginī. Photograph by the author, 2013. Associated with description on p. 15.

5 Kālī's Tongue. Devotional image used for alms collection. Photographed with permission of owner, Assam, India. Photograph by the author, 2013. Associated with description on p. 28

6 Kālī Mahāvidyā, Kālī the Great Wisdom. Original painting by Max Dashu, 2000, www.maxdashu.net. Used with permission. Associated with description on p. 50.

7 Offerings. Photograph by the author, 2013. Associated with description on p. 78.

8 The wild river Kālī has Aditi's head, at the Narmadā Kālī Temple near the Bhedaghat Yoginī Mandir, Madhya Pradesh. Photography by Durgadasi Devi, 2011. Used with permission.

*General Index

**See* Index of the Hundred Names of Adya Kālī, which follows General Index

A

abhaya mudrā, 143, 184, 217
adornment, 137, 177
Ādyā Kālī, about, 12-13, 15-18
Ādyā Pīṭh (Adya Peeth) temple, 15-18, 195
Ādyā Śakti, 196
alcohol, 75, 77, 78; *see also* nectar, wine
altar, *see* shrine
Ambuvācī (menstrual festival of the goddess), 52, 200, 217
amṛta (nectar), 110, 111, 137, 142, 144, 164, 169, 200; *see also* body fluids; nectar; sexual fluids
ānanda, 180
añjali mudrā, 75, 200
Annada Thakur, 15
āsana (seat), 69, 133, 145
āsana yoga, 38, 44, 200
ascension, as a spiritual path, 20, 47, 147
ascetics, asceticism, 42, 45
ash, 9, 143
Assam, India, 16, 18, 35, 51, 52, 67, 68, 119, 124, 151, 197, 200, 203, 217
Avalon, Arthur (aka Sir John Woodroffe), 83

B

Bande, 128
Barks, Coleman, 132
bells, Kālī's, 177, 178
belly, 10, 50, 115, 135, 136, 141, 146, 155, 156, 164; *see also* body
Bhairava, 55, 59, 129; *see also* Śiva, fierce
Bhairava Yāmala, 195
Bhairavī, 43, 59, 129; *see also* Daśa Mahāvidhyā (Bhairavī)
Biernacki, Loreliai, 52, 197
bījā mantra, 61-66, 76, 98-99, 100, 102, 180, 181-182, 185, 198, 200; *see also* mantra
bindu, 11-12, 52, 101, 151, 155, 179, 201; *see also* sindūr; tīlaka
birth/creation, 98, 142-143
bliss, 100, 117, 118, 157, 162, 180
blood, 138; *see also* menstruation; moon blood
body, 63, 117
  as temple/vessel, 25-26, 108
  imbued with practice, 138-138
  fluids, 11, 63, 111, 138-139; *see also* amṛta; nectar; sexual fluids
  nature of, 100
  of light, 14
  role in Kālī practices, 11, 21, 37, 46, 47-51, 52
  woman's sovereignty over, 53
bones, 9, 87, 138, 142-143
boredom, in spiritual practice, 68, 171
Brahma, 32
Brahman, 201
Brahmamayī, 12

Brahminy ducks, *see* cakravaka bird
breath/breathing, 70, 128, 135; *see also* prāṇayāma
Bṛhannīla Tantra, 57, 197
burning grounds, 9; *see also* cremation grounds; funeral pyre; ghāṭ

C

cakra, 4, 123, 145, 201
cakravāka bird (Brahminy ducks), 136-137
camphor/camphor offering, 90, 165-169
cared for, by Kālī, 172
causal body, 99-100; *see also* subtle body
celibate path, 129
challenges, offering to Kālī, 173, 174-175, 182-183
channels (in the subtle body), *see* nāḍi
Chinnamastā-Cāmuṇḍā, *see* Daśa Mahāvidyā (Chinnamastā-Cāmuṇḍā)
Chitgopekar, Nilima, 45, 46
commitment, to practice, 4-5, 61- 64, 70-74, 76, 78, 158, 161, 181, 183; *see also* vrata
community, *see* practice-community
compassion, *see* nectar, of compassion
constriction/closure, versus openness, 20, 22, 23, 24, 29, 102, 136
courage, 110
crone, *see* hag
cremation grounds, 8-9, 10, 59, 127, 143, 174; *see also* burning grounds; funeral pyre; ghāṭ
Cudala, 129

D

Dakini Lion-Face, 128
Dakṣiṇeśvar Temple, 15, 16, 17, 18, 193, 195
Dakṣiṇkālī, 12, 13, 17-18, 193
dance
  Kālī's, 9, 55-56, 122, 143
  ours, 114, 136, 139, 147
dark goddess, xi, xii, 10, 11, 32, 33, 34, 73, 99, 108, 191, 196, 203
darkness, 11
darśan, 15, 125, 131, 201
Daśa Mahāvidyā, 34, 50, 119, 196, 197, 201, 203, 209
  Bhairavī, 36, 68
  Chinnamastā-Cāmuṇḍā, 36
  Dhūmāvatī, 36
  Kālī Mahāvidyā, 36, 52, 62, 64, 216, 217
  Kāmākhyā Mahāvidyā, 52, 64; *see also* Kāmākhyā Goddess
  Ṣoḍaśī, 36
  Tārā, 36
Dasdatta, Ramlal, 8
Dashu, Max, 217
death, 9, 99, 100, 107, 134, 184-185
  accepting, 142-143
Delhi, 193
descent, 196,
desire, 50, 64, 103, 105, 128, 149-153, 182, 185, 203
  and Kāmarūpa, 118-120
  and Kulakāminī, 183-184
  and the Sixty-four Arts, 100-102
  /Desire, 38, 51-52, 120
  transformed, 130
Devī, 14, 19, 36, 37, 49, 83, 99, 104, 201
  and the Kumārī, 123-125
devotion, 64, 108, 114
Dhūmāvatī, *see* Daśa Mahāvidyā (Dhūmāvatī)
dhyāna, 158, 201
discipline, 68-70
dreadlocks (matted hair), *see* hair
dual awareness, 21-22, 29, 133
dual feminine, 34, 196, 202; *see also* jami (twins)
Dutt, M.N., 58

E

elements, *see* tattva
evil, 122, 182-183
eyes-covered practice, 118

F

fear/fears, 28
  of our mortality/death, 142, 184-185
  as offering, 147-149, 150
feast, *see* Tantric feast
feminine, 12; *see also* practitioner, mature female; yoginī/yogi
  as spirit—masculine as matter, 43

feminine *continued*
focus, of the Song practice, 97
fierce
deities, 30, 59, 117
desire, 47
forms of Śiva, 105, 106; *see also Bhairava*
goddesses, 10, 11, 32, 33, 52, 59, 99
fierceness, vii, 27, 46, 105, 106, 127, 134, 136, 193, 208
of Kālī; *see* Kālī, fierceness of
fire, of practice, 9, 108, 125, 130
and Kālī's different forms, 11, 84, 108, 114-115, 116, 166, 180, 186
in the subtle body, 114-115
of transformation, 27, 29, 50, 114-115
fish, 77
flower petals, *see* petals
fluids, *see* body fluids; sexual fluids
friends, spiritual, *see* gopī/Gopī; sakhī
funeral pyre, 9, 143; *see also* burning grounds; cremation grounds; ghāṭ

G

Gaṅgā, 174
Ganges river, 174
ganjā berries, 83, 199
garden, *see* jasmine garden; *see also* kadamba forest
garland, 4, 68, 78, 90, 132, 133, 143, 162; *see also* jasmine garland
of bone, 87, 143
of camphor, 90, 166, 168
of heads, 26
of letters, of the Sanskrit varṇa-mālā, 65
of kadamba flowers, 86, 132
gāyatrī mantra, 65; *see also* mantra
generative organs, 102-103, 111; *see also* yoni
ghāṭ, 174, 201; *see also* burning grounds; cremation grounds; funeral pyre
goddesses' (Kāmākhyā) scattered body parts, 119-120
"good student," 25
gopī/Gopī, 86, 127-131, 202, 204, 206; *see also* sakhī
Goudriaan, Teun, 17, 59, 197, 198
grace, 111-114
Guhya Kālī, iv
guru, 16, 17, 18, 45, 62, 77, 185, 202, 205
gurvī (female teacher), 18, 45, 62, 77, 172, 185, 202, 205
gynocentrism, 35-36, 41-46

H

hag, 18, 129, 135
hair, 24, 26, 50, 56, 105, 109, 121, 129, 162
matted (dreadlocks), 29, 72, 83, 84, 105, 109, 167
healing, 29, 44, 79-80, 125, 127, 164, 165, 180-181, 182
hibiscus, 76, 78, 143, 192
householder path, 129

I

identification with Kālī as deity, 104
intoxication, 138-139, 141, 146-147, 169
Inanna, 24, 196
iṣṭadevatā/ iṣṭadevī, 65, 202
"it's not happily ever after," 133-134

J

jami (twins), 34, 202; *see also* dual feminine
japa, 38, 65, 69, 158
jasmine
as offerings to Kālī, 26, 78, 131, 192
garden, 131, 132; *see also* kadamba forest
garland, 70, 143, 159, 162, 168
journaling/writing, 79, 100, 102, 103, 106, 127, 148, 181
joy, 173
Jvālāmukhī, 193

K

ka, 58, 184, 195
kadamba
flowers, 86, 132, 133, 134
forest, 86, 127-134, 136-137; *see also* jasmine garden
fruit, 138
wine, 138, 140, 141
Kaimal, Padma, 38

Kālī, 10, 11, 12, 57, 59, 77, 99, 122, 197
as darkness , 117-118, 120-121
as inseparable from the teaching, 172-173
as mother, 9, 10, 12, 17, 28, 37, 43, 54, 56, 127, 160, 163-164, 206
as dark mother, 10, 24
as fierce mother, 26
as mother of desire, 51, 119
as mother of time, 84, 72, 107
as womb mother, 14, 18
in mother-child relationship with devotees, 90, 163, 183-184
as primordial reality, 10, 12, 15, 49, 58, 98, 115
as primordial womb, 13, 14, 17, 18, 19, 59, 119, 145, 175
as ultimate reality, 12, 14, 15, 17, 195, 201; *see also* Kālī-Brahman
as womb goddess, 13, 14, 19, 49, 52, 107, 119
black like Kṛṣṇa, 116-117
cared for by, 172
central teaching of, 126
duality/paradox of, 9, 10-11, 12
fierceness of, xi, 8, 10, 11, 19-31, 32, 33, 99, 109-110, 111, 113, 117, 122, 148, 191; *see also* Bhairavī
her
lap, 169
love, 163
triangle of union, 142-143
identification with, 104
in love with, 5, 8, 9, 10, 18, 25-26, 31, 67-70, 73, 79
Mahāvidyā, *see* Daśa Mahāvidyā (Kālī Mahāvidyā)
names, using, 71-73; *see also* Index of the Hundred Names of Ādyā Kālī *which follows* General Index
-nityā, *see* nityā; moon phases
nourishing relationship to, 70-71
practitioner as, 3, 10, 11, 15, 97
pūjā, 3
tawny-colored, 115-116
transcendent nature of, 59
woman as, 43-44, 46, 50
Kālī-Brahman, 12
Kālīghāt, 193
Kālīkula, 5, 34, 48, 49, 50, 51, 59, 171-173, 196, 202-203
kāma (desire), 203; *see also* desire/Desire
Kāmākṣī, 119; *see also* Kāmākhyā
Kāmākhyā, 16, 68, 124, 197, 201, 217
as bindu, 51, 52, 64, 119, 151
and desire, 51-52, 64, 88, 120, 149-150, 151, 163,
Kāmākhyā as Kālī, Kālī as Kāmākhyā, 64, 119-120, 180, 182
Kāmākhyā as a yoni goddess, 18, 51-52
Kāmākhyā and the Daśa Mahāvidyā, 197, 201
Pīṭha, 88, 151
Kāmarūpa, 18, 88, 119, 120, 149, 150; *see also* Kāmākhyā
kapāla (skull cup), 130, 142-143, 203
Kāśī-Varanasi, 174, 175
Kathmandu, 193
kaula, 39, 93, 183-184, 196, 203
kaulika, 91, 93, 171, 172, 183
Kolkata, 15, 55, 198
Kṛṣṇa, 116-117, 127-130
kula (spiritual clan/family), 34, 50, 67, 171-172, 173, 184, 196, 203; *see also* Kālīkula; paramparā; practice-community
and kinship terms, 198
kulācāra (kula teachings), 171-172, 203
Kulārṇava Tantra, vii, 160
Kumārī, the virgin girls, 85, 123-127, 134, 165, 203
pūjā, 85, 123, 124, 125
kuṇḍalinī, 11, 109, 198

L

Lajjāgaurī, 13, 25, 195, 217
Lakshminkara, 128
Lal Ded, *see* Lalla
Lalleshwari, *see* Lalla
Lalitā, *see* Śrī Lalitā
Lalitā nityā, *see* nityā; moon phases
Lalitavajra, 128
lay practitioner; *see* householder path

Lalla, 128, 131-132
left-handed path, 196; *see also* Tantra/Tantric
life-force, *see* śakti-prāṇa
light of Kālī, 14
light versus dark, 20-21, 24
lilā, 55-56, 88, 101, 137, 151, 204
lineage, 30, 33, 34, 53-54, 57, 76
 of Kālīkula, 5, 35, 36, 41, 43, 48, 51, 97, 103, 106, 138
 Tantric, 23, 27-28, 38, 77, 118, 143
liturgy, of the names, 4-7, 11, 25, 31, 47, 51, 59, 78, 106, 156, 175
 mantric qualities of, 61, 65; *see also* mantra
 how to recite, 71-73, 185
lolling tongue, 28
Lopamudra, 128
lotus flower, symbolism of, 144-147
love-prāṇa, 141

M

McDaniel, June, 196
McDermott, Rachel Fell, 9, 12, 197
Mahākālī, 13, 58
Mahānirvāṇa Tantra, 5
Mahāvidyā, *see* Daśa Mahāvidyā
makāra (pañcamakāra/five offerings), 77-78, 156, 204
mālā (rosary), 65, 204
 of bone, 143
 of kadamba flowers, 132, 133, 134
maṇḍala, 50, 52, 79, 102, 140, 204
mantra, 38, 44, 61-66, 68-70, 135-136, 170-171, 205; *see also* bījā mantra
Mātṛkā (the mothers), 34, 52, 119, 196, 203, 204
meditation, 38, 136, 176
melancholy, 180
menstrual
 blood, 52, 196; *see also* moonblood
 festival of the Goddess; *see* Ambuvācī
menstruating Goddess, 47, 51, 52, 119, 200; *see also* Kāmākhyā
menstruation, 47, 48-49, 52, 196, 119-120; *see also* moonblood
mercy, 111-114
mind, Kālī overwhelms, 176-177
Mirabai, 128
moon, 10, 33, 34, 85, 121, 138, 179
 bright, 34
 crescent, 85, 121, 179
 dark, 26, 33, 34, 71, 131, 202
 full, 33
 new, 156
 phases, 33, 49, 101, 196; *see also* nityā
 moonblood, 25-26, 48, 51, 78, 107, 111, 196; *see also* menstrual blood; menstruation
Mother Kālī, *see* Kālī as mother
Mount Meru, 178, 179
mudrā, 75-76, 77, 160, 204; *see also* abhaya mudrā; añjali mudrā; yoni mudrā
mūrti, 16, 17, 52, 120, 205
musk deer, 164-165
musk/musk offering, 89, 90, 161-165

N

nāḍi/channels (in the subtle body), 100, 138, 141, 146, 155
Nathan, Leonard and Clinton Seely, 10, 19, 27, 43
nectar, 144, 164, 170; *see also* amṛta (nectar); body fluids; sexual fluids
 of compassion, 72, 84, 110-111, 113
 with camphor, 90, 168-169; *see also* camphor/camphor offering
 wine- , 86, 88, 90, 138-139, 140-143, 156-161, 168, 169; *see also* alcohol
New Delhi, *see* Delhi
nityā, 196; *see also* moon phases

O

offering/offerings, 44, 77-78, 107, 112, 120, 141
 "even when it's a stretch," 152-153
 five sacred, *see* makāra (pañcamakāra/five offerings)
 making/being, 161-162
openness, practicing, 20, 22-25, 29, 102, 108, 122-123, 174
oppression, 196

P

pañcamakāra, *see* makāra (pañcamakāra/five offerings)
paramparā, 59-60, 197, 205; *see also* kula
Pārvatī, 33, 127, 129, 130
Pashupatinath, 193
perfection, 79, 116, 186
petals, 3, 75, 144, 166, 198
Pīṭha, 205; *see also* Kāmākhyā Pīṭha; Sakta Pīṭha
play, sacred, *see* lilā
pleasure, 175
  finding in practice/sādhana, 168, 170
poetry/poems, 8-9, 9-10, 13-14, 19, 26-27, 43
polarity/polarities, 38, 103, 117, 149
pot, *see* womb pot; water jar
practice/practices, spiritual, 4, 11, 12, 21, 26, 27, 44, 70-71; *see also* sādhana
  as enactment of deity, 67
  deepening, 22-24
  community, 4-5, 6, 20, 25, 31, 34, 35, 44, 139, 202, 206; *see also* kula; paramparā
  in the kadamba forest, 131
  invisible, 31
  secret, 35, 38-39, 76, 109, 139, 164
  Tantric, 29-31, 33-35, 45, 59, 118
practitioner
  as deity, 38, 41, 44, 97, 159; *see also* Kālī, woman as
  mature female, 127-131, 133-134
  qualities needed, 31
prāṇa, *see* śakti-prāṇa
praṇām mantra, 65, 205; *see also* bījā mantra; mantra
prayer/prayers, 42, 75, 120, 158, 186-187
pride, 104-105, 106
pūjā, 36, 63, 156, 158, 161, 162, 166, 168, 170, 205, 208
  community Kālī Pūjā, 3,
  Kumārī Pūjā, 123-126; *see also* Kumārī
  morning after, 167
pyre, *see* funeral pyre

R

Rādhā-Kṛṣṇa, 17, 18
Rājarājeśvarī, 33; *see also* Śrī Lalitā; Sundarī; Tripurā Sundarī
Rāmakṛṣṇa, 15, 16, 195
"Renowned Goddess of Desire" (Kāmākhyā), 52, 119
relationality, 42, 63
resistance, 68-70
rest, 112-114, 125
retreat practice, 139-140, 150
  in darkness, 118
revision, your childhood, 124
rice, 75, 198
ritual, 75-77, 123, 124, 126, 142, 165; *see also* shrine
rosary, *see* mālā
Royal Asiatic Society of Bengal, 198
rūpā, 85, 120, 126, 149, 150, 205

S

sacred community, *see* practice-community
sacred play, *see* lilā
sādhana, 4, 35, 63, 64, 152, 180-181, 205; *see also* practice/practices, spiritual
  "not always pretty," 10, 25, 108, 110, 180
Śaivism/Śaivite, 32, 33, 39, 196, 206
sakhī, 63, 129-130, 133, 152, 198, 202, 205-206; *see also* gopī/Gopī
Śākta, 196, 198, 206
Śākta Pīṭha, 52, 119-120, 193, 196, 197, 206
Śakti/Śiva, 44-45, 132, 147
Śakti/śakti, 17, 32, 39, 53, 54-55, 149, 150, 198, 207
  and desire, 64
  meaning of 36-38
  -prāṇa (life-force), 48, 61, 146, 156, 198
  three aspects, 48; 51, 52
śaktipat, 198; *see* kuṇḍalinī
Śaktism, 33-34, 196
Śaktisaṇgama Tantra, 42, 197
sandhyā bhāṣā (twilight language), 36, 76, 77, 138, 160, 165, 207
saṅkalpa, 4, 158, 207
Sanskrit alphabet, 4, 58, 65

Schelling, Andrew, 20
secrecy
and Tantric practices, 38-39, 76, 150, 164
and women practitioners, 35, 76, 109
seed mantra/syllable, 61-66, 98; *see also* bījā mantra; mantra
Seely, Clinton, *see* Nathan, Leonard and Clinton Seely
self-care, 112, 127-128, 181
self-love, 31, 104, 115, 153, 177, 183
Sen, Ramprasad, 9, 26-27, 43
separation, delight in, 129
service, *see* seva
seva (service), 104-105, 207
sexual
desire, 103, 119, 141; *see also* desire
fluids, 111, 139; *see also* amṛta (nectar); body fluids; nectar
as nectar, amṛta, 111, 141, 144, 157, 164, 169, 200
union, 128-130; *see also* union
sexuality, on the spiritual path, xii, 14, 38, 50-51, 53, 54, 103
and abstinence, 28
shadow, 26, 170, 180
Shakya Devi, 128
Shaw, Miranda, 46
Shaza Khandro, 128
shrine, 4, 25, 26, 68, 120, 136, 140, 146; *see also* offering/offerings
creating, 44, 73-79, 142, 185
open-air, 12, 15-16
to Kāmākhyā, 51; *see also* Kāmākhyā
siddhi, 157-158, 207
sindūr, 76, 167, 207; *see also* tīlaka; bindu
sisterhood, *see* sakhī; gopī/Gopī; practice-community
Śiva, 9, 15, 32, 40, 105-106, 109
fierce forms, 105, 106; *see also* Bhairava
in relation to Kālī, 121-122
Sixty-four Arts, 100-102
sixty-fourth name, 161
skull cup, *see* kapāla
sloka, 197; *see also* stotra/stotram (hymn)
Ṣoḍaśī, *see* Daśa Mahāvidyā (Ṣoḍaśī)
spiritual family, 67-69; *see also* kula; paramparā
spiritual practices, *see* practice/practices, spiritual
Śrī (goddess), *see* Śrī Lalitā
Śrī Lalitā, 33, 34, 196; *see also* Rājarājeśvarī; Tripurā Sundarī
nityā, *see* nityā; moon phases
Śrī Rāmakṛṣṇa, 15, 16
Śrī Śāradā Devī, 15, 195
Sītā, 33
spiritual commitment; *see* saṅkalpa; vrata
Śrīkula, 33, 34
Śrīvidyā, 33, 196, 207
stotra/stotram (hymn), 100, 207; *see also* sloka
student, 25, 39, 62-63
subtle body, 16, 22, 69-70, 99-100, 112, 117, 130, 138, 145, 146, 155-156
suffering, vii, 22, 54, 68, 122, 134-136, 173, 174, 176
Sundarī, *see* Tripurā Sundarī
surrender, 68-69, 101, 104-105, 169, 182, 183
of habits/beliefs, 24, 28-29, 44

T

Tantra/Tantric, 62, 77-78
defined, 38-39
path, 27-29
practices, *see* practice/practices, spiritual, Tantric
practitioners, 199
Tantric Buddhism, 197
Tantric feast, 85, 125-126, 147, 156, 158, 204; *see also* makāra
Tantrik Hymn to Kālī, 5
Tārā
as one of the Daśa Mahāvidyā, 36
in Buddhism, 144
tattva, 14-15, 65, 207-208
teacher, 31, 39, 62-64, 67, 77, 78, 138; *see also* guru; gurvī
tenderness, 154-155
Thadani, Giti, 34, 196
Tibetan Buddhism, 197
tīlaka, 162, 208; *see also* bindu; sindūr
time, 25, 29, 57, 58, 112, 115, 116, 158

time *continued*
and space, taking, 22, 34, 111, 129, 135, 139, 181
devourer/mother of, 84, 106-107, 179
in the dark, 118
practice over, 66, 70-73, 77-78; *see also* practice/practices, spiritual; sādhana
transformation, 113, 135-136, 142-143
trauma, 53, 180, 181
Tripurā Sundarī (Tripurāsundarī), 33, 207; *see also* Rājarājeśvarī; Śrī Lalitā
twilight language, *see* sandhyā bhāṣā

U

ugrā, 27, 208
underworld, 24, 196
union, 104-105, 114, 133-134, 137, 142, 144-145, 147, 151, 176
and practice, 54, 63-64, 70, 71, 73, 123, 128, 129, 161, 173
and intoxication, 138-139, 157, 162, 167-168
in/through the body, 11, 46, 47, 77, 109, 111
of the dualities, 34, 38-40, 103, 110, 117, 122, 143, 149
sexual, 129-130, 163-164
/Union, 51, 120
yoga of, 49, 65, 66, 130

V

Vaiṣṇava, 208
Vaiṣṇavism, 32-33, 39, 208
Vajrayana, 197
varṇa mālā, 208
Varanasi, *see* Kāśī-Varanasi
Viṣṇu, 32
vow; *see* saṅkalpa; vrata
vrata (vow/promise/spiritual commitment), 62, 160-161, 208-209

W

water jar/pot, 39; *see also* womb pot
winds (in the subtle body), 100, 155
wine-nectar, *see* nectar, wine-
wisdom goddesses, *see* Daśa Mahāvidyā
wisdom stream, 62-63
womb, 34, 47-49, 58, 59, 97, 115, 122, 136, 145
as seat of power, 102, 107
-aspect, 10, 12, 13, 14, 17, 18, 24, 25
-pot, 74-77, 148, 198, 217
women, 35, 41-44, 45-46, 123-127; *see also* feminine; Kumārī; practitioner, mature female; yoginī
Woodroffe, Sir John, *see* Avalon, Arthur
wounding, 26, 52-53, 120, 122, 127, 170, 180-181, 182

Y

Yāmala, 59, 195, 197-198
yantra, 179, 198, 209
Yid Trogma, 128
yoga, 49, 53, 54, 65, 66
of union, *see* union, yoga of
yoginī/yogi, vii, 4, 97, 138, 143, 155, 160, 199
accomplished/mature, 129-130, 131, 133-134
defined, 21, 53, 160
initiation from, 45-46
wandering, 185
with waist bells, 178
Yoginī Temple, 25
Yoginīs, the, 52, 59, 101-102, 119, 193
yoni, 13, 30, 130, 209
cleft of Kāmākhyā, 51, 52, 120
-crucible, 74, 75, 113, 114, 115, 130, 140, 141, 148, 158
-goddess, *see* Kāmākhyā; Lajjāgaurī; Kālī as womb goddess
- maṇḍala, 50, 209; *see also* yoni-yantra
-mudrā, 75-76, 160, 209, 217
-nectar, 144; *see also* amṛta (nectar); body fluids; sexual fluids
- pīṭha, 52, 119, 151, 209
-pot, *see* womb pot
-womb-, 35, 48, 49, 53, 97, 107, 109, 113, 115, 122, 146, 155
-yantra, 13, 209; *see also* yoni-maṇḍala
Yoni Tantra, 50
yoni triangulation, 113, 185
Yonigahvara Tantra, 59, 143

Index of the Hundred Names of Adya Kālī

Kadambapuṣpamālinī (35), 86, 133
Kadambapuṣpasantoṣā (34), 86, 132
Kādambarīpānaratā (39), 86, 138
Kādambarīpriyā (40), 86, 140-141
Kadambavanasañcārā (32), 86, 127-128, 130-131
Kadambavanavāsinī (33), 86, 131-132
Kādambinī (25), 19, 85, 120-121
Kalādhārā (26), 85, 121-122
Kalahaṃsagatiḥ (47), 87, 147
Kalakaṇṭhā (37), 86, 135-136
Kālakaṇṭakaghātinī (100), 93, 184
Kalamañjīracaraṇā (91), 92, 177
Kālamātā (9), 72, 84, 107
Kalanādaninādinī (38) 86, 136-138
Kālānalasamadyutiḥ (10), 72, 84, 108-109
Kālarātriḥ (22), 19, 85, 117-118
Kalāvatī (4), 71, 83, 100-102
Kālī (1), 71, 83, 98; *see also* General Index
Kalidarpaghnī (6), 71, 83, 104-105
Kālikā (8), 72, 84, 106-107
Kalikalmaṣanāśinī (27), 85, 122
Kalpalatā (53), 88, 152-153
Kalyāṇī (3), 71, 83, 99, 100
Kāmabījajapānandā (95), 93, 180
Kāmabījasvarūpiṇī (96), 93, 181-182
Kamalā (5), 71, 83, 102-103, 105
Kamalālayamadhyasthā (45), 87, 145
Kamalāmodamodinī (46), 87, 146-147
Kamalāsanasantuṣṭā (43), 87, 144
Kamalāsanavāsinī (44), 87, 144-145
Kamanīyā (52), 88, 151
Kamanīyaguṇārādhyā (55), 88, 154
Kamanīyavibhūṣaṇā (54), 88, 153
Kāmapāśavimocinī (24), 85, 120
Kāmapīṭhavilāsinī (51), 88, 151
Kāmarūpā (23), 85, 118-120, 149
Kāmarūpakṛtāvāsā (50), 88, 150
Kāmarūpiṇī (49), 87, 149
Kāñcanācalakaumudī (94), 92, 179
Kāñcanādrikṛtāgārā (93), 92, 178
Kaṅkālamālyadhāriṇī (42), 87, 143
Kapālapātraniratā (41), 87, 142-143
Kapardinī (11), 72, 84, 109
Kapardīśakṛpānvitā (7), 72, 84, 105
Kapilā (19), 84, 115-116, 137
Karālāsyā (12), 72, 109-110, 113
Karālī (2), 71, 83, 98-99
Kāraṇāmṛtasantoṣā (58), 88, 156-157
Kāraṇānandajāpeṣṭā (60), 89, 158-159
Kāraṇānandasiddhidā (59), 88, 157-158
Kāraṇārcanaharṣitā (61), 89, 159

Kāraṇārṇavasammagnā (62), 89, 159-160
Kāraṇavratapālinī (63), 89, 160-161
Karpūracandanokṣitā (73), 90, 167
Karpūrakāraṇāhlādā (74), 90, 168
Karpūramālābharaṇā (72), 90, 166-167
Karpūrāmodamoditā (71), 90, 165-166
Karpūrāmṛtapāyinī (75), 90, 168
Karpūrasāgarālayā (77), 90, 169
Karpūrasāgarasnātā (76), 90, 169
Karuṇāmṛtasāgarā (13), 72, 84, 110-111
Kāśīśavaradāyinī (88), 91, 175
Kāśīśvarakṛtāmodā (89), 92, 175-176
Kāśīśvaramanoramā (90), 92, 176-177
Kāśīśvarī (86), 91, 174
Kaṣṭahartrī (87), 91, 174-175
Kastūrībhojanaprītā (70), 90, 165
Kastūrīdāhajananī (68), 90, 163-164
Kastūrīmṛgatoṣiṇī (69), 90, 164-165
Kastūrīpūjakapriyā (67), 89, 163
Kastūrīpūjanaratā (66), 89, 162-163
Kastūrīsaurabhāmodā (64), 89, 161-162
Kastūrītilakojjvalā (65), 89, 162
Kaulikapriyakāriṇī (82), 91, 172
Kaulikārādhyā (81), 91, 171-172
Kautukinī (84), 91, 173
Kiśorī (36), 86, 134-135
Klaibyanāśinī (48), 87, 147-148, 149
Komalāṅgī (56), 88, 154-155
Kṛpādhārā (15), 84, 113-114
Kṛpāgamā (17), 84, 115
Kṛpāmayī (14), 84, 111-112, 113
Kṛpāpārā (16), 84, 113-114
Kṛśānuḥ (18) 84, 114-115, 116
Kṛṣṇā (20), 84, 116-117, 128
Kṛṣṇānandavivarddhinī (21), 84, 117
Kṛśodarī (57), 88, 155-156
Kulācārā (83), 91, 171-172
Kulakāminī (99), 93, 183-184
Kulamārgapradarśinī (85), 91, 173
Kulīnā (80), 91, 171
Kulīnārtināśinī (98), 93, 183
Kumārībhojanānandā (30), 85, 125-126
Kumārīpūjakālayā (29), 85, 124-125
Kumārīpūjanaprītā (28), 85, 123-124
Kumārīrūpadhāriṇī (31), 85, 126-127
Kumatighnī (97), 93, 182-183
Kūrcabījajapaprītā (78), 91, 170
Kūrcajāpaparāyaṇā (79), 91, 170-171
Kvaṇatkāñcīvibhūṣaṇā (92), 178

About the Author

ADITI DEVI began the study and practice of South Asian Tantric traditions more than twenty-four years ago. As an initiated yoginī, pujarini (ritualist), and lineage holder, she has lived and practiced her sādhana with adepts in Nepal, India, and Tibet. Aditi's practice, teaching, research, and writing focus on the embodiment of the divine feminine in the Śākta Tantric traditions of India and Nepal. She is authorized to teach the Kālī Practices focusing on the reverence of women as embodiments of the divine and awakening in the body, in deep relationality. These practices have their fullest expression in Assam, at the Kāmākhyā, one of Aditi's spiritual homes and practice seats. She is also a scholar of Tantra, and earned a Ph.D. in Anthropology, and was a Fulbright scholar and college professor before turning full-time towards the ways of the yoginī.

After several years of living in a remote contemplative community, Aditi has taken to the wandering life again, bringing her offerings to yoga retreats, teacher training courses, festivals, godowns, and wherever yoginīs and yogins gather. She recently returned from pilgrimage in India where she followed the trail of fierce desire, visiting several remote Yogini Temples.

When not wandering, Aditi Devi Ma's teaching home is in the foothills of the Rocky Mountains, where, she teaches privately, offers regular Kūlī Pūjā and Kirtan, yoga and meditation, and has established The Shala: A Classical Tantric Mystery School for Yoginīs and Yogins. She is also a faculty member at the Integral Center in Boulder.

Contact Information: www.aditidevi.com

About Hohm Press

HOHM PRESS is committed to publishing books that provide readers with alternatives to the materialistic values of the current culture, and promote self-awareness, the recognition of interdependence, and compassion. Our subject areas include parenting, transpersonal psychology, religious studies, women's studies, the arts and poetry.

Contact Information: Hohm Press, PO Box 4410, Chino Valley, Arizona, 86323; USA; 800-381-2700, or 928-636-3331; email: hppublisher@cableone.net

Visit our website at www.hohmpress.com

CPSIA information can be obtained
at www.ICGtesting.com
Printed in the USA
FSOW03n0341111016
25888FS

9 781935 387541